Blow the House Down

The Story of My Double Lung Transplant

Charles Tolchin

Writers Club Press
San Jose New York Lincoln Shanghai

Blow the House Down
The Story of My Double Lung Transplant

Published by Writers Club Press
an imprint of iUniverse.com, Inc.

For information address:
iUniverse.com, Inc.
620 North 48th Street
Suite 201
Lincoln, NE 68504-3467
www.iuniverse.com

ISBN: 0-595-00558-6

Printed in the United States of America

Dedication

Dedicated to my donor
My donor was a seventh-grader named Valerie. She died
at the hands of a hit-and-run drunk driver. In their
worst hour, she and her family saved my life.

Contents

List of Illustrations

❀

Acknowledgments

I am deeply indebted to my family and friends who edited this manuscript. Through their insights, they each helped shaped this book. Editors include: Susan Tolchin, Martin Tolchin, Karen Tolchin, Eve Jaffe, Dr. Linda Paradowski, Jonathan Markowitz, Steve Brown, Stu Cowan, John Hale, David Hilzenrath, Phil Saltzman, Amy Kaden, Joan Weiss, Judith Benkendorf and Michael Copperman.

I would also like to thank the Fairfax County, VA, Park Authority, for allowing the use of the Mt. Vernon Recreation Center Ice Rink for the cover photograph.

Cover photograph: Joe Connors

Introduction

On April 13, 1997, I got a phone call. It came at 6:18 in the morning. Before I picked the receiver up from its cradle, I looked at the digital clock on my dresser and I knew what was coming. For twenty-eight months, I had been on the waiting list for a double lung transplant. For the past five, I had been number one.

A chain of events had now been set into motion that would forever change my life.

CHAPTER 1

❀

Growing up with Cystic Fibrosis

Sometimes I get goose bumps when I think of how my life has changed. They come at random moments, like when I'm stopped at a traffic light in my old neighborhood, when I'm walking my dog in the park, or when I'm riding up the elevator at work. At those moments, I am struck by an incredible thought: I have new lungs. This is the story of how I came to receive them.

Before my lung disease took on a more prominent role, my life was full of promise. Slowly, over the course of years, I went from being a normal, active kid, to a teenager who spent weeks at a time in the hospital. Still, I graduated from college and began a career in advertising.

Then, my health abruptly halted my career and called into question the promise of my early years. A double lung transplant offered the only hope I had.

The experience would force me to fight hard.

Now, my new lungs enable me to once again lead the normal, healthy life that I had been forced to put on hold at a young age. They enable me to pick up the adventure right where I left off.

My transplant began with a conversation in May of 1993. Dr. Sandra Walden worked at Johns Hopkins University Hospital, in Baltimore, Maryland and treated adults who had Cystic Fibrosis. With free-flowing hair and funky skirts, she looked like a throwback to the seventies.

She treated me for CF, a disease that affects the lungs and digestive system. The disease clogged the small airways of my lungs with mucous and made them like large sponges dipped in honey. This genetic defect led to frequent infections.

When I met with Dr. Walden, I was twenty-four years old, lived in Richmond, Virginia, and worked in advertising for Circuit City. It was my first job after college, and I had just progressed from "new clueless guy" to "new guy who's starting to hit his stride."

Weeks earlier, I had gotten sick. As is routine with CF patients, the bacteria that colonized in my lungs had raged out of control. This required two weeks of IV antibiotics to stem the infection. From the age of 16 on, I have usually required this at least once a year.

My parents, Susan and Martin, dropped everything in their own lives and drove down from their home in Bethesda, Maryland. They picked me up in Richmond and took me to Hopkins. At the end of my two-week stay in the hospital, Dr. Walden told me that I had recovered well. But then, as I sat in an orange plastic chair, she told me that I should start thinking about a double lung transplant.

This floored me. I was completely surprised that anyone would think that I needed a transplant. Even with only 30% percent lung function, I thought I was too healthy. In fact, I had grown up considering myself that way. When I was a small child, my baby-sitter broke her ankle trying to keep up with me. In elementary school and junior high, I played soccer. Back then, I had been completely unhindered by my illness. Health was only a minor factor. I caught colds more often than other kids, and sometimes I coughed hard. But I went camping, played in the mud, and served on the safety patrol.

In high school, I played on the tennis team, served as class president, went to Daytona Beach with my friends, and in general, found very creative ways to be wild and not get in trouble. It was a blast.

In my mind, I was still that normal person. I was not someone who was so sick that he needed a transplant. Dr. Walden's assessment jarred my self-identity.

That normal demeanor was instilled in me by my parents. They let me go to sleep away camp. They allowed me to ski in harsh weather, do karate, and go sailing. They let me grow up thinking that I was normal.

My mom is a professor of public policy at George Mason University. My dad is a journalist. He spent 40 years at the New York Times, then founded his own paper, The Hill. Together they have written six books that explore disturbing aspects of government policy. My sister, Karen, is two years younger. She is beautiful and witty. She hopes to become an English professor. As a family we are loving, upper-middle-class, and hard working.

My parents got news of my diagnosis when I was five. I cannot imagine the thoughts that ran through their heads. I only know what they were told: my life expectancy was eight years of age and that there would never be a cure. For me, the experience is a vague memory of tests. Being a typical kindergartner, the only part that I remember with clarity is that one day the hospital staffers had a big white sheet-cake for a celebration and gave me a piece. I do not remember ever being specifically told that I had CF.

After I was diagnosed, my parents pushed on, fighting hard to find the best medical care possible. They found the best doctors, the best medicine, and the best treatments. They learned about CF research, and fought with every resource they had, to get more funding for it. It is through their example that I learned tenacity.

Fighting is the one core tenet that has propelled me in life. It is what I cling to when I am stripped down and have nothing else. It is my survival default when I must act on pure, primal instinct. It is almost as though I have been programmed to think this way in moments when rational or conscious thought is beyond me.

Transplant had been suggested to me once before, in 1987 by Dr. Beryl Rosenstein, who managed the pediatric CF practice at Hopkins. He bore an air of warmth about him and smiled the way some people do when they are totally comfortable in their own skin.

Dr. Rosenstein had admitted me to the hospital for a two-week course of antibiotics. CF had always been a kids' disease, but because of all of the research breakthroughs, adults with CF were becoming a new phenomenon. We were however, often treated by pediatricians, and when admitted to the hospital, placed on children's wards. When I was admitted to Hopkins in 1987, I stayed on a ward that consisted mostly of young people. There I met patients who had problems far worse than CF: three and four-year-olds with leukemia, bald from chemotherapy but happily tugging their IV poles in front of them as they walked; a thirteen-year-old boy who had his legs blown off by accident on his farm, and had miraculously dragged himself over fields to get help; a beautiful young woman about my age, a tennis coach, who had a severe case of Lupus. I learned from all of them. Those young people gave me strong sense of perspective.

At the end of my stay at Hopkins, Dr. Rosenstein suggested that I may need a lung transplant within the next few years. I disagreed with him, and did not think about it too much, and basically shrugged it off. I did not feel that sick. Unlike when Dr. Rosenstein broached the subject of transplant, now I believed Dr. Walden.

After I returned to Richmond, I thought hard about Dr. Walden's comment. My main concern was that if it was time to start thinking about a transplant, then I certainly was not doing everything that I could do to stay healthy. If I did indeed decide to work harder at staying healthy, a massive amount of time would be required on my part. Would I have to leave Circuit City to dedicate my time to my health? I considered my career precious. Would I be forced to throw it away? Would I go crazy if I was unable to work in advertising?

If I did spend more time on my health, what exactly did that entail? With CF, there are a number of treatments that patients can do at home to clear the thick mucous from their chest. With postural drainage, a care giver cups his hands and claps in a rhythmic motion on the chest, back and sides of the person with CF. The cupped hands produce sound waves that vibrate through the lungs and mechanically shake the mucous loose so that it can be coughed up. Gravity is also used to help. The patient changes positions, sometimes lying on a table in a head-down tilt. A treatment takes between 30 and 45 minutes.

This is sometimes referred to as "chest PT," short for physical therapy because the treatment is usually performed by physical or respiratory therapists. Nurses, parents, wives, siblings, and baby sitters also perform chest PT. My parents diligently did chest PT on me for years, beginning when I was diagnosed.

I have a number of friends who have successfully used it as an entre to sex with their girlfriends. It's physical and there's a convenient flat surface.

A second way to loosen the mucous is by inhaling nebulized medicine. Usually it is a mixture of bronchodialators and saline. Other medicines can be done as well. This takes about fifteen minutes per treatment.

As I thought about taking better care of myself, I wondered whether or not I should do more chest PT and nebulizing. I could not do it more than twice a day and still work full time. The same could be said for dedicating more time to lifting weights and exercising.

Leaving Richmond would be incredibly hard. I loved my job so much. I had ascended through the rough part of the learning curve and was finally hitting my stride at work. I did not want to give that up. My apartment was becoming a real home. I loved locking the front door at

night and having my own space. And I loved Richmond with its barbecue joints, eclectic undercurrents, and Southern pace.

I did not want to abandon the normal life that I led.

A small coterie of medical professionals offered advice including Dr.
Chernick and Dr. Rosenstein. I knew other people had been in my situation before, and I wanted to know what they did. One person who
was especially helpful was Joanne Alford, a clinical nurse who worked
for Dr. Rosenstein up in Baltimore. I called her one day during my
lunch hour from a pay phone in the lobby of my office. We had a very
long conversation. She didn't tell me to take an action one way or the
other. But she told me what other patients had done and what their
experiences had been.

In the few weeks during which I struggled to decide, eleven friends of
mine who had CF died. A number of my friends had died from CF over
the years, but never such a dramatic number in such a short time period.

Jason Corallo's death was the worst. Jason used to lift weights with
me. He was thin and wiry, and had the comedic air of Don Knotts. He
also had a very healthy sexual drive. If he saw a beautiful woman driving
along in traffic, he would follow her to the nearest gas station, get out of
his blue Dodge Daytona, and introduce himself. Jason and I had both
received chest pt from an attractive respiratory therapist named Donna
Haas. When Donna arrived at Jason's house one day, his grandmother
opened the door, took one look at her and exclaimed: "Now I know why
Jason looks forward to chest pt all of a sudden."

Jason was sicker than many people. He had received IV antibiotics
frequently enough to merit a portacath, a permanent IV connection
lodged in his chest. People get those for two reasons. The most common
reason involves peripheral IVs, or those in the arms. After getting IVs
repeatedly, a vein cannot be accessed any more. Eventually, all of the
veins in both arms reach that condition. A second reason is one of
patient preference. Some patients don't like being stuck all the time. IVs
need to be removed after about three days and restarted in another site

to prevent an infection from brewing in the vein. If a person knows that he will be receiving IV's four times a year, and he blows a vein every two days, that can add up. Some people decide to spare themselves the hassle. With a portacath, the use of needles becomes obsolete. With his portacath in place, Jason never wavered in the gym, even when doing the bench press.

One day I got a phone call from Jason's mother, Leslie. I had never met her in person so I knew something must be wrong if she was calling. She told me that Jason had gotten very depressed. He stopped eating, taking his medicine and doing chest pt. As a result, his health deteriorated rapidly.

He locked himself in his room and refused to see anyone. Jason and I had originally met when a physical therapist named Frank Duchesne introduced us. Jason idolized Frank. Frank was handsome, athletic and a perfect older brother type. Jason refused to see Frank. He refused to see Donna. All of our CF friends were frantically beating the jungle drums, trying to find a way to reach him. We failed miserably. Jason died within a week. Most people with CF do not die like him.

Most people fight very hard to stay alive. My friend Nanette Anderson stands out as an example of that drive. She was petite, blond, and devoutly religious. Like me, she hung out with a large pack of friends. To the untrained eye, she bore no resemblance to a U.S. Marine or pro-football player. But the courage and grit she demonstrated far eclipses what most of us could even imagine.

At the time when she went into cardiac arrest, she was already in the hospital. The doctors that were trying to save her put her on a hand-held ventilator and were squeezing the bag to force air into her lungs. Nanette reached out and compressed the bag harder and faster because she knew she was dying and the people trying to save her were not fighting hard enough.

I miss Nanette and Jason and think of them often.

According to Dr. Milica Chernick of the NIH, most CF patients die
of cardiac arrest as a secondary effect of pulmonary failure. The lungs
fail to provide enough oxygen to the heart.

Dr. Chernick had been my doctor since the eighth grade. She grew up
in Macedonia. That communist upbringing translated into modest
tastes and an air of humility. Like the character Yoda in Star Wars, Dr.
Chernick combines a very unassuming appearance with deep brilliance
and insight. She is a trainer of Jedi Warriors. Over the years, she has
become a true friend and a member of our family.

As a physician, Dr. Chernick offers deep compassion to her
patients. Having a lung disease means an endless procession of cold
stethoscopes on one's chest. Dr. Chernick always made sure to warm
hers before taking a listen.

I regret terribly the fact that I didn't travel up from Richmond to try
and see Jason. I should have camped out on the other side of his door
and just talked through the wood until I annoyed him to the point
where he would respond. But because I had missed so much work from
being in the hospital, I couldn't drop everything. And because I had gotten sick so quickly, I wanted to use my weekends to stay put and rest up,
not run back and forth to Maryland, get exhausted and sick again.

Jason's death, along with those of my other ten friends, highlighted
for me the importance of my health. It served as a flashing, neon bill-
board that read: "Wake up, you idiot." In retrospect, I think it also
stressed the importance of control. To me, being sick meant no control.
I wanted to regain that.

Shortly after Jason passed away, I went into my boss's office and
resigned.

When Kim Mathis, who worked over in the creative department, heard
the news, she had a unique reaction. We had become friends, having
lunch once now and then, and going to the occasional party together. She
came with me to a CF fundraiser downtown earlier in the Spring.

When she learned of my departure, she invited me over to her apartment for dinner. Kim was half Italian, so I suspected she might be a very good cook. That was not the case. She made a lasagna that tasted God-awful. The noodles were soggy, and the contents consisted only of rancid cheese and tepid sauce. There was no meat or spinach. Actually, the food didn't really matter. We had a really good conversation.

Kim combined a cosmopolitan stylishness with a strong sense of independence. She had long red hair and a face that belied her thoughts far too easily.

At the end of our dinner, Kim expressed to me her feelings about my resignation. She told me that she was really upset because she had a huge crush on me. Things progressed from there.

Before I left that evening, she insisted that I take home all of the leftover lasagna. I didn't want to insult her, so finally I accepted it. It took a week to get the rank smell out of my car. Our friendship turned passionate and my final six weeks in Richmond were the best because of her. On the last night I spent in Richmond, she put on a white cocktail dress and took me out for a big steak dinner.

Chapter 2

Taking Control of My Health

Moving back to my parents' home made me feel like a complete failure. I had to rent out a mini-storage unit for all of the furniture from my apartment. I had to move back into my old bedroom. And at the age of twenty-four, I had to resume the role of a dependent. Up until this point, I had led a fairly normal life, filled with exercise, friends, dating, college and working. Now, my path would deviate.

To avoid going crazy, I engaged in a number of activities.

I began doing a small amount of marketing consulting. First I did some work for a friend. She was in the process of starting up a new business importing white asparagus from Peru. Later, I consulted for a growing chain of bicycle stores, Bikes USA.

I also began to seriously write. When I was in college studying business, I loved listening to the stories of successful companies. I thought they were heart-warming. Wouldn't it be a good idea, I thought, to write business-oriented stories for kids? Now I had the time.

A friend, Amy Goldberg, had recently moved back to the area and taught fourth grade nearby. We first met in seventh grade and have remained friends ever since. She has flowing red hair and down-to-Earth values. From seventh grade until senior year of high school, she dragged a large pack of us to each horror movie that came out. She loved hard-shelled crabs and talking on the phone.

Amy invited me to read my work to her class. The students had a very positive reaction. As a result, I wrote more. My sister, Karen, became a wonderful mentor in this regard. Things had gone sour with a boyfriend in Harrisburg, Pennsylvania, and she moved back to Bethesda. She finished writing a fine novel of her own, *The First Jewish Viking*. It was a coming of age narrative set at Bryn Mawr. Karen showed me that a real-live young person could set out to write a novel and complete it. In my eyes, she made a very lofty goal achievable.

***

Now that I was living at home, I dedicated a great deal of time to taking care of myself. I began to do my respiratory therapy routine three times a day.

First I would nebulize a bronchodilator for twenty minutes. With my small airways opened up, I would then nebulize Pulmozyme for twenty minutes. Pulmozyme, or DNAse, was designed to thin the thick mucous that plugged my small airways. Researchers had learned that the CF mucous contained long chains of white blood cells that helped it thicken. The drug was designed to cut those long chains, thereby thinning the mucous.

DNAse entered into phase three clinical trials halfway through my senior year of college at George Washington University. I enrolled as a participant in the study at Johns Hopkins University. The study was double-blind, which meant that neither the doctors nor I knew if I was actually receiving the medicine. The study was very time intensive. It meant two twenty minute nebulizer treatments every day. It meant frequent pulmonary function tests in Baltimore. The first week of the study, I had to travel to Baltimore three times for pulmonary function tests. After that, it was once a week.

After using Pulmozyme, I used the ThAirapy Vest for half an hour to cough out the loosened mucous. The Vest enabled me to stop meeting with a physical therapist every day. This was incredibly liberating. Ever since the beginning in my senior year of high school, eight years earlier when Dr. Chernick recommended it, I had been receiving professional chest PT every day.

The Vest negated the need to coordinate with a therapist seven days a week. It lowered the cost of my care considerably. And I could treat myself more than once a day. The machine consisted of a vinyl vest connected to an air compressor. The air flowed into the vest in rhythmic pulses. Instead of a pair of hands clapping one side of me at a time, I now had a machine percussing all sides of me at once. Just like with a physical therapist, I used my Vest on a tilt-table. This enabled me to change sides, thereby draining the mucous from all lobes.

The Vest made me cough like crazy and proved to be very effective at clearing out mucous. No longer did I have to coordinate my schedule with a therapist. No longer did I have to wait if they were caught in traffic or delayed by other patients. Now I could do more than one treatment a day if I so desired. Within the confines of my life, it was liberating.

There were two drawbacks to the Vest. First, the air compressor weighed one hundred and ten pounds, which made it hard to transport. The second drawback was that it was very loud, and sounded like a jet engine revving up for takeoff.

The final step in my routine involved the Flutter. It was a small, handheld device that I blew into. It basically simulated the effect of exhaling hard through pursed lips. The Flutter had a steel bal! bearing inside. When I blew into the Flutter, the force of my breath pushed the ball up and down a fraction of an inch, very fast. The vibration sent a backwave of pressure down into my lungs that helped loosen more mucous.

With my last treatment of the day before bed, I skipped the Pulmozyme portion of my regimen. Most people only use Pulmozyme once a day, but Dr. Chernick felt that I could benefit from a second dose. Each dose cost twenty-nine dollars.

My respiratory therapy routine sapped a massive amount of time out of my life. On average, I spent about five hours a day doing nebs, the Vest, and the Flutter. Added to that, I worked out at least four times a week for an hour or two. Most afternoons, I needed to nap for an hour or two. And I spent an exorbitant amount of time eating six or seven times a day. This basically left one or two hours to get things accomplished.

I became totally obsessed with my time, and hated doing things like going to the Motor Vehicle Administration. That in itself could take all of my free time for the day. I hated going to the doctor because no matter where I went, they made me wait. The thought of missing a session of chest PT for that reason made me cringe.

Getting out of the house in the morning became a feat. Chest PT and nebs took almost two hours. Adding in breakfast, a shower, and walking my dog, Bogart, I was looking at three hours. If I woke up at eight a.m., that meant not being ready for the day until eleven. By that point, it was too late to go to the gym because I would never complete a workout before lunch.

Working out was very important. During my freshman year of high school, my body was fairly scrawny. I weighed one hundred and twenty pounds and stood five feet tall. That was not surprising because malnutrition is the norm among people with CF. We cannot digest food properly, and our hearts and lungs have to work harder than normal. This creates a very high metabolism where we burn up every calorie we ingest. Dr. Chernick gave me some advice that miraculously sunk into my brain. She sat me down in her office on Ward 9D at NIH and told me that "I was at an age where I had the power to change how I looked." She encouraged me to build up my body by lifting weights and eating more.

Many of my friends played junior varsity football that year, and engaged in weight lifting. They brought me with them to workout with the football team during the off season, and in so doing, taught me the basics of the sport.

The football team's bare weight room consisted of rutted, mocha-colored tile walls, a floor covered with thick black rubber, naugahyde-padded benches, squat racks, and steel plates. There were no mirrors, posters, hot tubs or saunas. There was no music. There were no women. Just the hovering smell of pubescent sweat blended with the unfocused ambition of second-rate athletes.

We concentrated on two lifts: the bench press and the squat. For the first few months, I had no idea there were any other exercises. Most of the guys lifted hundreds of pounds at a time. They achieved this by placing 45 pound plates on a 45 pound bar. When I began, I could only bench press the bar with a ten pound plate on each side. I could barely remove a 45 pound plate if someone left it on the bar when they finished. Surprisingly, none of the football players looked down on me for my weakness. In fact, they respected me for applying myself and sticking to it. At that point I learned a vital lesson about weight lifting: everybody starts somewhere, and everybody progresses at his own pace.

One day, the wrestling coach spied me working out with the football team and tried to recruit me. With my light weight and rising strength, I could be a real asset to the team. I declined because I did not want to immerse myself in a culture that valued keeping weight down. I wanted to build mine up.

Weight lifting offered me a new world of positive role models. My friends and I worshipped Arnold Schwarzennegger. We watched all of his movies, *The Terminator*, *Commando*, and *Raw Deal*. *Conan the Barbarian* and *Conan the Destroyer* made especially large impacts. We still ask each other: "What is best in life?" and repeat Conan's response in Arnold's thick Austrian accent: "To crush your enemies, see them driven before you, and hear the lamentations of their women." When my sister, Karen, was a sophomore in high school, she often studied at American University's library. One day, walking through the reading room, she heard two college guys posing the question to each other. She stopped dead in her tracks, offered the "crush your enemies" line, and left them smitten.

The movie *Pumping Iron* about professional body building also added to our respect for Arnold. We used to recite his line about the "pump," or endorphin high he received while working out: "The pump is like the coming. I am pumped twenty-four hours a day. I am coming, twenty-four hours a day."

Arnold offered me a glimpse at the kind of body Doctor Chernick prescribed when she told me I had the power to change my appearance. I studied Arnold's physique and knew what pectorals were supposed to look like. The same with his deltoids, trapezeus, triceps and biceps. He gave me a body to aspire towards.

Weight lifting taught me valuable lessons in discipline. The first month that I began the sport, I remember being so sore from doing squats that I could barely walk up stairs. I saw no difference in the size of my muscles, but kept at it. Only very slowly did the changes emerge in my body. Dramatic changes in strength and muscularity would be years in the making.

Halfway through my senior year, I achieved a real milestone, I bench pressed one hundred and thirty-five pounds. This was significant to me for two reasons. First, to lift that, I had to lift the forty-five pound bar with two forty-five pound plates. When I started lifting, I could barely lift just one plate. Second, I could now bench press my own weight, a sign of strength.

***

In addition to weight lifting, I had to learn how to eat properly. People with CF can't digest fat so as soon as I was diagnosed, I had to start taking enzymes. Like all small kids with CF, the enzymes were a major fight. Back then, enzymes came in a powder form that was sprinkled directly on the food and made it taste disgusting. As a person who always loved food, this was simply unacceptable. Thanks to medical research, the powder soon progressed to pills and alleviated the problem.

In 1988, I took a year off of college to work for the CF Foundation. I helped the organization start a national, mail-order, discount pharmacy for people with CF. A year after opening our doors, we operated at a revenue level of $5 million per year. Today, the pharmacy is thriving, with annual revenue of $30 million and forty employees. It is the largest seller of many CF drugs, especially digestive enzymes.

During that year, I gained new insight into how to gain weight. I started the year still weighing one hundred and thirty-five pounds. For some reason, I had a flashback to my friend, Mike Simpson, in high school. He was always eating. During study hall at ten a.m., he whipped out a sandwich and chowed down when the teacher, wasn't looking. I thought that maybe if I ate six or seven times a day, I could gain weight. So in addition to my usual breakfast, lunch, afternoon snack and dinner, I began to weave in a mid-morning snack and a bedtime snack. Sometimes I consumed two afternoon snacks, eating at two p.m. and five, then dinner at seven.

In addition to eating more meals, I learned how to space them apart to stretch out my eating day. If I ate breakfast first thing when I woke up and had my last snack right before I went to bed, then that gave me more time to digest between meals. Keeping food available became very important. I always kept food in my desk, and I kept the kitchen well stocked. Never having to hunt for food made eating frequently so much easier. There were always onion bagels, boxes of peanut butter crackers, and frozen pizzas on hand.

I wanted to supplement my diet with high calorie milk shakes, so I went to the local supermarket and walked up and down the dietary supplement aisle, reading every label. I bought a six pack of chocolate flavored Ensure Plus, which had the most bang for the buck, 355 calories in an eight ounce can. Ensure became a staple of my diet, and I always kept a can in my desk and another in my golf bag. Soon I began getting creative with Ensure. I would dump it in a blender, along with a few scoops of ice cream. Then I would add whatever else might be on hand, Hershey's chocolate syrup, honey, or raspberry jelly.

I believe eating was important, but I had to give those calories somewhere to go. I continued weightlifting hard, and I could see the results working in tandem with my new diet. In a few months, I had gained thirty pounds, up to one hundred and sixty-four. Finally, Dr. Chernick told me not to gain any more, that it would be too much of a strain on my heart.

✶✶✶

Even with all of this additional respiratory therapy and regular exercise, I got sick soon after returning to Maryland in 1993. I needed IV antibiotics twice more by November. That would make four times since March. This was very unusual for me. Normally, I needed IV's once a year or so. Twice at the most.

Since my junior year of high school, I had slowly become accustomed to receiving antibiotics because I knew how much better I would feel at the end of the treatment. Each time took its toll on me however, as I began to feel like a wild beast being roped into captivity. I imagined myself literally being lassoed limb by limb.

My family was always very supportive, visiting me every day. My first few stays in the hospital, I could not stand the food. So Mom cooked for me at home and brought me lunches and dinners every day. At first she thought I was being a bit demanding. But then one day, she happened to be in my room when lunch arrived, a glop of reeking mush under a yellow plastic warmer. After that, she not only understood, but grilled the hospital dieticians.

My first admission to the hospital, in 1985, was very difficult for me. I was at an age where it was difficult to drop everything in my life. I missed two weeks of class. I missed two weeks of the varsity tennis team's season, for which I played doubles. I missed a Drug and Alcohol Awareness Day that I conceived and developed. I disappeared on my girlfriend for two weeks and did not tell her where I went.

My friends offered their support, visiting me en masse. The nurses had never seen a patient receive twenty rowdy teenage visitors at a time. They did not come quietly or unobtrusively. Mike Copperman would visit and then wander off to explore other parts of the hospital. He was especially drawn to the psychiatric ward. J.T. Jacoby would head straight for the patient refrigerator and indulge his healthy appetite. Others would help themselves to the phone and the television. Jon Hefter visited me every day without fail.

The one thing I hated more than anything was my friends and family seeing me in the hospital. I knew no matter what I did, it would be an image of me that they would never shake.

Other aspects of the hospital, however, proved highly enlightening. One of my closest friends dating back to Kindergarten is Mike Simpson. His dad, Bob, was a prominent researcher at NIH. Growing up, he had taken Mike and me camping and sailing. Bob once visited me in the hospital, and offered me very useful advice. He told me that if he were me, he would learn everything he could about CF. Those words would ultimately help me in my fight.

During that first hospitalization in 1985, I worked with a respiratory therapist named Mr. Davis. He was huge, over six feet two, came from Lake Charles, Louisiana, and had served as a medic in Vietnam. He told colorful stories and we got to be good friends. Every day, Mr. Davis would hand me a small hand-held spirometer, or pulmonary function test machine, and have me blow. Each day while on IV antibiotics, I could see improvement. When I left the hospital, I felt tremendously better. The antibiotics worked quickly and cleared up my infection. My lungs had much less mucous clogging my small airways and my pulmonary function improved. I coughed much less often.

***

When I began looking into transplant programs, I consulted the experts. Bob Beall was President of the CF Foundation. I had met him the summer after my freshman year of college, when I took a job as a communications intern at the Cystic Fibrosis Foundation along with four other CF adults from around the country. As an intern, I wrote for their national publication and I wrote congressional testimony. In the process, I learned a lot about CF. My internship began my fulfillment of Bob Simpson's advice.

It was during that internship that I first heard about the concept of transplantation as a cure. Suzanne Tomlinson served as consumer affairs coordinator for the Foundation, and we got to be good friends. One day, I was sitting on the orange-yarn sofa in her office, talking shop, when we received word that doctors had performed the first successful heart-lung transplant on a CF patient. We both felt like Tevye from *Fiddler on the Roof*: "May God bless and keep transplant far away from us."

Back then, the CF Foundation was run by Bob Dresing and Bob Beall. Bob Dresing served as president of the Foundation. He wore tortoiseshell framed glasses and dark suits, and exuded the air of a mid-western executive. He first got involved with the Foundation because his son, Rob, has CF. Parents like Bob form the backbone of the organization, infusing it with a sense of zealous urgency. Because their children have CF, they want to find a cure as soon as possible. Bob's dedication to the cause led him to leave his successful furniture retailing business and move from Ohio to Maryland so that he could be completely involved in the Foundation.

Bob Beall, then the Foundation's Medical Director, has a balding, blond pate and a flushed complexion. He is the quintessential type-A personality, the Tasmanian Devil in seersucker. Although he is not a parent of a kid with CF, you would never know it. He has channeled his energy and dynamism to unraveling the mysteries of this disease.

These are the men you want fighting to cure your disease. Under Bob Dresing's fund-raising direction, the Foundation went from raising fifteen million dollars a year for research up to sixty. He brought corporate management to a ragtag volunteer organization. He designed and branded events, and then launched them across the country. Because of Bob, events like our golf tournaments and walk-a-thons now had a professional, consistent quality to them. The people who attended them were sure to have a great time. Bob Beall directed the investment of that money. He hosted conferences that brought together the best medical minds, and he developed a network of premier CF care centers and CF research centers around the country. Together, Bob Dresing and Bob Beall lit quite a fire.

Together, they proved that good science can be bought. In 1989, Foundation-sponsored scientists Francis Collins, Lap-Chee Tsui, and Jack Riordan discovered the gene that causes CF. Throughout my entire lifetime, doctors had predicted that would never happen. A genetic breakthrough had been considered pure science fiction. As a child, however, I was never told this. As an adult, I never believed it. Luckily, those skeptics were proved wrong.

As an intern at the Foundation, I listened to Bob Beall and Bob Dresing speak about progress in CF research. They spoke with great confidence that in the not-too-distant future, there would be a cure for CF. They described in detail the process of the disease. And they spoke with great urgency, saying that the dollars could not come quickly enough. They had the power to inspire me towards a life of philanthropy. Nothing, it seemed to me, could be more important than investing in medical research and keeping scientists working hard on CF.

When it came time to look for a good transplant program, not exactly a category in the Yellow Pages, I sought Bob's advice. He had risen to become President of the Foundation. Bob told me that both Pittsburgh and UNC were first rate, but he gave UNC a slight edge. Washington University in St. Louis and Stanford out in California were the only other programs in this country of that caliber. Outside of this country, England had developed and perfected lung transplant. For years, their survival statistics were far better than the best centers in America and nobody could understand why. It turned out, the British were far more aggressive in their follow-up care post transplant. The moment a patient had a problem, they treated it. Once the Americans learned how to follow-up, their numbers caught up with the British.

Two friends of mine had undergone double lung transplants. Leslie Wells was one of the first. His was an incredible story. He was on full life support in the intensive care unit at NIH. The ICU doctors wanted to pull the plug. The medical ethicists concurred, feeling that he was costing too much money. But Dr. Chernick fought fiercely to keep him alive. Miraculously, Leslie got healthy enough to come off life support and fly to England, the only place they were doing transplants at the time. He paid cash, got new lungs, and is now healthy, married, and loving life ten years later.

Tom Faraday got his new lungs at Pittsburgh. He too, went through a dramatic metamorphosis. The last time I saw him before his transplant, he looked awful. He was severely underweight, which was made even more apparent by his height. On his six foot two frame, he had only one hundred and twelve pounds. He was in the hospital when I saw him, lying on his bed half asleep in a darkened room. An air of exhaustion seemed to drape over him like a well-worn hospital blanket. Two years later, I saw him again. This time I was in the hospital, and he stopped by to say hello. This was during my fourth hospitalization of the year. Tom was an entirely different person. He was a life force, radiant, smiling, full of energy and enthusiasm. He was tan from playing football and cycling, and now weighed one hundred and fifty pounds. He had married one of his respiratory therapists and he had gone back to work full time. He told me all about his transplant. He said there was no pain involved. I didn't believe him, but the thought of pain didn't bother me. He told me that he was in the hospital for five weeks after his transplant, and he told me how vigorous exercise after the operation built up his strength.

Dr. Chernick and Dr. Rosenstein both provided the same assessment about UNC. While Pittsburgh received more organs, UNC proved to have just a scootch more expertise. That was all I had to hear.

***

At that point, I went down to meet the lung transplant team at the University of North Carolina in Chapel Hill. The transplant coordinator was a nurse named Ellen Cairns. She was my connection to the program and we spoke on the phone. She scheduled the appointment and told me that they would want me to have an x-ray and an exercise test.

I flew into Raleigh/ Durham International Airport, rented a car, and checked into my room at the Hampton Inn Hotel. The Hampton Inn was located near the hospital, nestled among a grove of pine trees. During the twenty minute drive from the airport, I noticed that pines blanketed the entire region. I rolled down the car window and inhaled their rich scent.

Being totally obsessed about my chest PT, I had scheduled my flight so that I could do my afternoon respiratory therapy right after lunch and then head South. I wouldn't be able to bring my Vest on the plane because it weighed so much, so I would miss my evening treatment. I still did my nebulizer and doubled the time I spent with the Flutter. I

had scheduled old-fashioned chest PT in the physical therapy department at UNC the next morning, and hopefully, I would be home by
mid-afternoon in time for my next treatment.

When I got to the hotel, I realized that I had forgotten to pack one
crucial item: saline to mix in with my bronchodilator for nebulizing. In
a panic, I called Ellen at the hospital but she had already left for the day.
So I went to a nearby pharmacy and explained the situation to the
pharmacist. She told me not to worry. I could use contact lens saline
solution. It was identical to what I inhaled in my nebulizer.

After averting that crisis, I went out to dinner with Rachel Burnett.
Rachel and I had met my freshman year of college at Duke University in
an introductory psychology class. While I scraped by with a "D," Rachel
went on to earn a Ph.D. in the field. As always, Rachel was very supportive and we had fun together. During that dinner, she outlined the best
ways to pick-up women. She does not recall this topic of conversation.

The next morning, I began my sojourn into the world of transplant.

The University of North Carolina Memorial Hospital is a cutting-
edge medical facility in the middle of nowhere. One would expect such
a fine facility to be located in the heart of New York or Boston, cities
with considerable medical talent pools and rich supplies of wealthy
patients. But UNC grew to prominence despite its location, treating the
rural poor and the exploding population of the Triangle, the area
formed by Raleigh, Durham and Chapel Hill.

I had last been to UNC as a sophomore in college. Back then, I had
gone to receive treatment at the outpatient CF clinic. The facility looked
relatively similar, except that a few new buildings had been added to the
medical center. The eight story tower still rose above the main entrance.
The parking deck still lay across Manning drive, connected by a partially covered walkway. A helicopter pad lay between the two. New
research facilities had sprouted up as had a new Neurosciences building

and the Anderson Pavilion. The older parts of the hospital still stretched back behind the tower and to its flanks.

That morning, I scarfed down three Egg McMuffins and then headed to the hospital. I parked in the big deck, and walked across the partially covered walkway. A cluster of smokers with IV poles hung out just in front of the main entrance, a sight repeated outside of hospitals across the country. It never fails to sadden me how these people, no matter how ill, must feed their addiction. I held my breath and walked through the cloudy air to enter a hospital.

I wound my way through the halls and found the physical therapy department. A tech in the physical therapy department pounded on my chest. It was the first time a person had pounded on me ever since I switched to the Vest a year and a half earlier. He was very tall and thin and had a thick Boston accent. He had black hair combed straight back.

The physical therapy department plays an enormous role in the transplant team. Before Dr. Tom Egan, the head surgeon on the transplant team, decided to move to UNC and build a lung transplantation department, he rigorously interviewed the physical therapists. Were they interested in providing the massive amount of care he would demand of them? Their positive answers resounded.

The walls of the PT department enshrine the real story of transplant. Taped to the yellow-painted cinder block walls, posters donated by each graduate of the program motivate future patients. Some posters are of hunky guys, others are of athletes, some are inspirational, and some are just quirky. Each poster is signed by the person who donated it, and dated with the day they received new lungs. Their spirit radiates from the images they offer. That spirit spoke loud and clear: "ordinary people go through this with a sense of humor and live to tell about it. You can too." I did not even think that someday, I might contribute a poster to this collage. It seemed too far away, too abstract.

After he finished pounding on me, Mike introduced me to two patients who were waiting for new lungs. They came to "pulmonary rehabilitation" in the PT department three times a week to exercise on the stairmasters, treadmills, and stationary bikes. This built up their strength for the operation. Patients who had recently received new lungs came to PT later in the day and worked out four times a week. At rehab, the therapists monitored the patients' pulse-ox, or pulse and the amount of oxygen in their blood. They also kept a notebook on each patient, detailing the extent of each workout.

I chatted with the two patients, a young man and a young woman. The woman had CF but the young man did not. Neither seemed nervous in the least bit. To the contrary, they badly wanted to receive their new lungs. Both of them had moved to Chapel Hill at the request of the transplant team so that they could be nearby when their organs became available.

After a few minutes, a physical therapist took me on an exercise test. The exercise test is used by the transplant team to determine endurance. The patient walks as fast as he or she can for six minutes on a predesignated course through the halls of the hospital. The physical therapist monitors the patient the entire time with a hand-held pulse-ox machine.

I did well on the exercise test, jogging for part of the way. The therapist who monitored me struggled to keep up with me, and at the end of six minutes, complained that the bursitis in her hip flared up. That made me very proud. In six minutes, I covered eighteen hundred feet.

Next I went to x-ray. At this point in my life, I had been x-rayed many times. I stood with my chest against the cold metal, took in a deep breath and held it, then breathed. Automatically and without instruction from the tech, I turned to align my left side against the machine and I raised my arms to hold the bar above. I felt like Nicholas Cage in *Raising Arizona*, a repeat offender well familiar with mug shot procedure.

Finally, I went to the transplant clinic. Seeing the sign for "Cardiothoracic Surgery" made me a little nervous. The words themselves sounded highly invasive. The waiting room had a bluish-green carpet and lighting that muted the white walls. The room was crowded with other patients, all mixed together from different clinics.

First I met Ellen Cairns. She had a mop of dark brown hair and freckled cheeks. She went over my vital signs, the medicines I was taking, and my history. Then I met Dr. Tom Egan. He was a surgeon, the first I ever met. He had a big smile, a thick black mustache, and a pack of five residents following closely behind him. Two character traits became immediately apparent: curiosity and bluntness.

Dr. Egan told me that I was not ready for transplantation because I was not sick enough. "You are far better with your own lungs than with anyone else's, so you should try to keep them as long as possible," he said. He told me that I was too healthy even to go on the waiting list. He explained how they tried to time transplantation down to when a person probably had about a year or less to live. It was very difficult to predict. He said that the pulmonary function test of FEV1, forced expiratory volume in one second, was the most important number they looked at. An FEV1 below thirty percent meant that it was time. Mine was right about thirty. He told me that he had one patient who was a big racquetball player. When he couldn't play racquetball anymore, that's when he knew it was time for transplant.

Dr. Egan told me about the survival rate for double lung transplant at UNC. He said that only five percent of the patients don't make it off the table. At the one year mark, ninety percent were still alive. After that, it decreased ten percent a year, down to fifty percent survival at five years. This didn't bother me because I knew that if you needed a transplant, those numbers beat the hell out of your odds if you didn't receive one. I knew also that the numbers encompassed a broad range of patients, some of whom were very sick at the time of their operations, while others were healthy. I knew that I would be strong at the time of my transplant which would give me a significant advantage.

Dr. Egan was glad I checked in with them when I did, well before I needed a transplant. He told me that many people come to them once they get sick and consequently have a difficult time waiting. At that point, he told me that the waiting time for new lungs was eighteen months to two years.

Before Dr. Egan left, he told me to come back in four months for a check up. Then he asked if I had any questions for him. "Do you have any advice for someone like me?" I queried, not sure of even what to ask. "Keep healthy and keep your insurance," he replied without missing a beat.

On my way back to the airport, I realized that during my two hour visit at UNC, not one person took a listen to my lungs with a stethoscope. I was surprised, but to me, it was apparent that they knew what they were doing. I decided to not even meet with the transplant surgeons at Pittsburgh.

CHAPTER 3

❀

Life in Limbo

When I returned to Maryland, my life was in a strange limbo. I wasn't waiting for a transplant, but I was waiting for the time when I might be. I had a limited amount of free time, and a vast amount of captive time doing respiratory therapy. I knew that I had to keep my mind active, so I began writing in greater detail.

Karen had written a wonderful novel, so maybe I should take a stab at it. With that in mind, I began to write a thriller. I had always liked mysteries and thrillers, and had grown up reading Agatha Christie, Robert Ludlum, and my favorite: Ken Follett. At Duke, one of the few courses that I enjoyed was a course in mystery fiction taught by a wayward grad student and attended mostly by second semester seniors.

What topic did I know enough about? The life that I missed terribly: advertising. By spending my days in a fictional advertising agency, I could at least taste my former life and the one I aspired towards again someday. I could create imaginary conversations between account executives and agency presidents. I could carry on great marketing debates.

I could talk with art directors and copywriters. I completed *Dominant Influence* in about four months. It was about an evil ad executive who tries to sell tortilla chips in a very sinister manner.

Karen was a wonderful mentor, patiently editing each chapter as I pulled it off my printer. She taught me many of the basics of fiction writing: how to describe a person; how to create a character; how to find my voice. The book was weak, but I learned a great deal in the process. Karen and I began to develop our own lingo about writing, and our own strong opinions about what seemed to work and what did not.

Writing was a good avocation in that I could do it while I inhaled a nebulizer treatment. I could write while laying on my tilt-table with my head down, connected to the Vest. In fact, I always kept a legal pad and felt-tipped pens on top of the washing machine next to the table. I quickly learned the importance of keeping more than one pen on hand: frequently, I would drop a pen by accident, and with an extra, I didn't have to unhook myself from the Vest, climb down from the table and retrieve it. I had to use felt-tipped pens because ball-points, which I normally prefer, do not work for long upside down, the position I wrote in.

***

In addition to my writing, a few people went out of their way to keep me connected with the world. Each time they called or invited me out, they let me know that they cared about me. They broke up the monotony in my life and helped me experience some semblance of a normal social life. I know that helped preserve my sanity.

Amy Goldberg had moved back to Maryland after a three year stint teaching disadvantaged fourth graders in San Antonio, Texas. This was the first time the two of us lived in the same city since we had graduated from high school. We soon began a ritual every Wednesday night: a big group of us would get together for a potluck dinner. Then we would watch *Beverly Hills 90210* and *Melrose Place*. I was usually the only guy in attendance and therefore loving life.

Mike Taylor and I met in seventh grade home room. We went on to share a locker throughout all four years of high school. Mike graduated from law school and started his own general practice in Rockville, Maryland. He and I went to lunch often. If I listed our favorite culinary destinations, one might question my dedication to healthy living. Needless to say, more than a few calories were consumed.

My cousin Jonathan Markowitz in Chicago went far out of his way to keep me connected to the world. We joke that "Cousin Jonnie from Chicago" sounds like a Mafia nickname, but he's actually on the up and up. Jonathan has a seat on the Chicago Mercantile Exchange and is the managing partner in his commodities trading company. He is slightly eccentric in that his mind constantly zings from one idea or opinion to the next. He is balding, has a goatee, and smiles with his eyes.

Cousin Jonathan sent me a modem. I installed it myself, and went on-line. From that point on, I spent countless hours e-mailing friends around the country, staying in touch.

Jonathan did something else that boosted my self-esteem. He regularly asked for my help in writing and editing various documents. While it may seem trivial, it actually made me feel as if I were contributing to society in some way. During this period in my life, I got a real sense that my friends did not want to burden me with their problems. I felt as if I couldn't be there for them, or help them when they needed it, and that made me very sad. People like Amy Goldberg, Mike Taylor and Cousin Jonathan all shared their problems, and I am grateful.

Kim Mathis also made me feel connected. We stayed in touch and saw each other every other month or so. Usually, I would drive down to Richmond for a day to see her. I didn't want to stay longer because that would mean missing a Vest treatment. She lived in a third-floor walk-up, and hauling the Vest up those stairs would have been a feat. But we wrote to each other and spoke on the phone regularly, and she made me feel that I wasn't a loser.

In March of that year, Aaron Roffwarg got married. He first burst onto my scene when I was four years old, on Cape Cod, Massachusetts, in a small town called Wellfleet.

Because of his propensity towards mischief, Aaron's sister, Anna, referred to him as "Devil Child."

Karen and I boarded on a plane and flew to Houston for the festivities. I brought my flutter and my nebulizer, but could not bring my ThAirapy Vest. I felt naked without it for three days, but Dr. Chernick assured me that I would be fine with the Flutter. Aaron had offered to find a physical therapist for me, but that was not necessary.

***

To heed Bob Simpson's advice that I should learn everything I could about my health, I now had to learn about transplant.

Kim Brown helped in that regard, having received three kidney transplants. Kim grew up in Denver, smelled of floral perfume, and was quick to laugh in a rapid fire staccato. She worked in the United States Capitol for the Sergeant-at-Arms. She described for me her experience with transplant and became a good mentor.

Kim was involved in a transplant organization, TRIO, Transplant Recipients International Organization. She encouraged me to attend their events, which I did. There I got to meet a cross-section of transplant recipients: heart, kidney, liver, and a few lungs. Lungs were rare, though.

Like Kim, the other recipients were warm, friendly, and informative. They ranged in age from the young to the old, and comprised a broad socio-economic and multicultural range. They did not carry themselves as people who had walked through fire. They were modest. Even so, their sense of resilience shone through.

***

During the year, I returned to Chapel Hill every four months for a check up. I got to meet a number of the pulmonary residents, and on one visit, I met Dr. Linda Paradowski, the head non-surgeon on the transplant team. In the classic childrens' book *The Lion, The Witch and the Wardrobe,* there is a character named Mrs. Beaver. When four children are lost in a scary forest and pursued by an evil queen and her secret police, Mrs. Beaver takes them into her home, cooks them "a great and gloriously sticky marmelade roll," and warms them up. Dr. Paradowski was cut from that same mold. You know that if you were wandering around a scary forest, she would take you in and warm you up.

Dr. Paradowski had short, gray hair, attractively styled. She stood with her hands stuffed in the pockets of her black slacks, and emitted a modesty very similar to Dr. Chernick. When I met her, I had just finished up in clinic, and was crossing the waiting room to leave. She was out there chatting with a patient, Brian Urbanek. He had recently received new lungs, but he did not look well. His face was slightly swollen from steroids. He was slouched in a chair and looked a little down in the dumps. Dr. Paradowski and Brian told me that transplant wasn't always smooth sailing. Apparently, he had problems with rejection. For some reason, this didn't scare me. I just assumed that would not be the case when my time rolled around.

On my next visit to UNC, I saw the face of smooth sailing. Her name was Monica Goretski. She was beautiful and carried herself with a casual poise, confident and happy as she worked her way across the waiting room. There was only one quality about her that clued me in to the fact that she had a transplant. She had a look in her eyes that many Vietnam veterans get, one of complete fearlessness and stoicism. I wish I could have spoken with her but I was too shy to approach her. I did, however, remember her, and burned her image in my memory as a positive transplant role model. Much in the way Arnold Schwarzennegger served that purpose for my weight lifting, Monica's example set the tone for how I wanted to go through my transplant. I wanted smooth sailing.

I wanted to walk through the waiting room a year later with my head
held high and a laid-back, no-worries air about me, just like her.

On my return trips to Chapel Hill, I got into the same pattern of taking a late-afternoon flight, renting a car, and staying at the Hampton
Inn. I also reconnected with Annette Mortick, an amazing friend from
Duke. We had met our first night at Duke, at "Sue and Jim's China Inn,"
a dive famous for its lenient alcohol policy two blocks away. She was living two flights above me in Hanes Annex so her freshman orientation
group had gone out for Chinese food with mine. Since the food didn't
come for a few hours, we had plenty of time to realize that we had a lot
in common.

Annette was from Olney, Maryland, about twenty minutes away
from Bethesda. Her high school, Sherwood, fomented a rivalry with
Walter Johnson. Annette had run hurdles on the Sherwood track team.
She was tall, had a big smile, and took immense pleasure in giving me a
hard time. For the most part, she teased me about being lazy, especially
when I would call her from my basement room in the dorm instead of
walking up two flights of stairs to see her.

***

Two events occurred in the May of that year that had an effect on my
transplant. First, my father retired after 40 years at *The New York Times*.
Actually, he didn't stop working for a minute. He founded a newspaper
all about Congress.

Dad went through the entire process of starting a business. He rented
out office space, bought computers, and hired a staff of twenty-eight
people. He hired a designer to help create the look of the new publication, and he gave it a name: *The Hill*. To his credit, at a time in one's life
when most people put themselves out to pasture on the golf course, he
started working harder than ever. He learned the intricacies of printing,
distribution, and advertising sales. In September, he published his first

issue and it made quite a splash. *The Hill's* advertising revenue slowly built up, and the reporters broke a number of national news stories.

***

The second event that May involved Amy Goldberg. Amy took an active role in her students' lives. If they had a basketball game on a Saturday afternoon, she would go and root for them. If they had a soccer game, she would be on the sidelines, cheering away. Once in a while, I would go with her.

One sunny Saturday afternoon in May, she took me with her to watch her kids play soccer. During the second quarter, she tilted her face up to the sun and declared how much she loved summertime. Amy had always loved summer, spending her days life guarding and her nights going to Jimmy Buffett concerts.

At the very moment when she reaffirmed her affection for the impending solstice, I was struck by a powerful thought: ice-hockey. I'm not sure why, but I suspect it was from watching the soccer players run up and down the field the way hockey players skate up and down the ice. I had never been a huge hockey fan, although I rooted for the Washington Capitals. I had never played ice-hockey, only street hockey a few times back in high school. I hadn't skated in years. But all of a sudden, this thought filled my brain. I had to play. I felt like Richard Dreyfuss in *Close Encounters of the Third Kind*. He becomes obsessed with Devil's Tower in Wyoming to the point where he builds a muddy replica of it inside his house.

Amy told me to shut up. I was being a complete idiot. But that night, she changed her mind. We were out at a party on Capitol Hill and struck up a conversation with two young men. They said they played hockey together. Amy and I looked at each other, unable to ignore the coincidence. They gave me a phone number to call and I was on my way to slamming people into the plexiglass.

There was an adult hockey school for beginners sponsored by Hockey North America. A few weeks after calling for information, I went and scouted a summer league game to see if it was realistic for me to play. I had never seen amateur hockey, only professional, and that night I stood alone in the bleachers watching ordinary people have a great time. I knew I could do it, and wanted to hit the ice as soon as possible.

The league told me that the next school session would probably begin around November. My team would go through school together and then be placed in a league of other beginners. They would teach us hockey skating and the basics of the game. All summer, I looked forward to hockey school. In the fall, I bought a pair of skates and hit the ice for the first time. I wanted to get into hockey shape before school started.

Skating was incredibly hard. When I started, I could barely make it around the rink once before I had to stop and rest. My shins killed me. I struggled to maintain my balance. For some reason, I was not deterred. I kept at it and slowly got a little better. Now I could skate around the rink twice before I had to rest. I went out and bought a complete set of hockey gear: shoulder pads, helmet, pants, gloves, elbow pads, sticks, tape, puck and a bag to carry it all.

✳✳✳

Getting an agent or publisher interested in *Dominant Influence* proved to be a challenge, so I started writing a second novel. This would be different than my first one. I would take longer to think about it, structure it with more plot elegance, and write it. I would create better characters. I would also make it a true mystery, solvable by the reader.

As I began to plot out my new novel, the things I learned from *Dominant Influence* served as a real springboard. I set my mystery in a New York advertising agency. Instead of trying to sell tortilla chips, I centered the story around the advertising of athletic shoes. It led me to the novel's true innovation: the heroine, an advertising executive, uses market research tools like focus groups and surveys to solve the crime. That had never been done before and I got very excited about it.

✳✳✳

In October I got sick and had to go to the hospital. My last course of IVs had been the prior November. I was pleased that my health had stabilized. It was clear though, that it now took much more effort to stay healthy compared to when I lived in Richmond.

After I left the hospital, I went down to UNC for a routine check-up from the transplant team. There I met with a pulmonologist on the team named Robert Aris. He had classic features, handsome eyes, and black hair that fused a fifties pompadour with eighties blow drying. He checked me out, and then stepped outside of the exam room for a moment. He returned with Ellen Cairns. That's when I realized something might be out of the ordinary. They both sat down and Dr. Aris told me that he wanted to do a thorough, three day long evaluation for transplant on me. Ellen would work out the details. Before the three-day evaluation, he wanted me to get two more weeks of IVs so that I could be in the best shape possible. I didn't think that was necessary because I knew I was in very good shape. My PFT's had recovered, my weight was good, and I felt strong. However, I was scared to give the transplant team the impression that I might be difficult. I feared that they might not get me new lungs if I constantly questioned every decision they made. So I called Dr. Chernick from Raleigh/ Durham Airport before I boarded my plane and arranged with her for another two week stay in the hospital.

✳✳✳

Something terrible happened during that second course of IVs. Dr. Chernick gave me the same antibiotics I received two weeks earlier, Tobramycin and Pipercillin. However, after a day, I had an allergic

reaction to Pipercillin that sent me into near shock. I got severely nauseous, weak, and my blood pressure dropped very low. I also got severe
myalgia, or pain, in my legs to the point where I could not stand up.

This was puzzling and at first, Dr. Chernick did not know what
caused it. She tried to give me the same medicine a second time under
her close supervision. She stood next to me and chatted with my parents as the medicine infused. Thirty minutes into it, I knew the reaction
was starting again. This time, she took my blood pressure every five
minutes and my blood every twenty minutes. The blood pressure cuff
hurt very badly. It felt as if it were squeezing the life out of my arm. This
was a replication of the myalgia in my legs. She started cranking me full
of fluid at a rate of 500 cc's an hour. After a few hours, I stabilized and
Dr. Chernick relaxed.

The nurses on the floor, however, did not relax. They thought I
would need more care than they could provide, and asked that I be sent
to the intensive care unit for observation. This made me very nervous.
I had never been to an ICU before. The ICU doctors came down and
told me it wouldn't be bad at all. I made them promise that they
wouldn't put an arterial line in my wrist to constantly measure blood
gases, and I made them promise not to put in a urinary catheter. On
both counts, they grudgingly agreed.

I was wheeled up to the ICU, met a very attractive nurse named
Belinda, and began to calm down. I forced myself to urinate as often as
possible just so that there would be no doubt as to the fact that I did not
merit a catheter.

After I settled in up in the ICU, Mom and Dad left, as did Dr.
Chernick. Then an unfortunate thing happened. Grandma tried to
call me in my old room. A respiratory therapist named Carl was in
there changing the tubing on my nebulizer and for some reason, felt
compelled to answer the phone. Carl wore his hair in a long pony tail
and had a tattoo on his forearm depicting his favorite brand of ciga-
rette rolling paper. He had a very colorful past. He was not the typical

lung-care professional, but I liked him a great deal. He was anti-establishment, a George Carlin-type contrarian.

Carl did not realize that my grandmother had a heart condition and a great capacity for worrying. So he told her that I had just been moved up to the ICU. She of course went into a full-panic, convinced that the family was hiding information from her. Calming her down was quite a feat, and I don't think my mom has forgiven Carl ever since.

I slept very little that night, but by morning, I had recovered. The ICU doctors released me back to the regular ward. There, I focused hard on recuperating. After a week and a half, my health was back to where it was when I was admitted to the hospital.

Dr. Chernick and the ICU doctors were stumped as to what caused my reaction to Pipercillin. They had the entire lot of Pipercillin checked out for contaminants but tests failed to surface any. They consulted with the Center for Disease Control and Prevention. They dug through heaps of medical literature, but on all counts, came up with nothing.

After the incident, I did not look back. I was just extremely grateful to be healthy once again.

CHAPTER 4

Placed on the Waiting List

Soon after being discharged from NIH, I headed back to UNC for a three day evaluation at UNC. This would answer a number of questions for the transplant team. First of all, it would tell them if I were in fact ready for a transplant. Second, if I were ready for a transplant, this would provide valuable information for them to use during surgery.

The transplant team told me that I would need to bring my family members with me during the evaluation. They wanted to be certain that I had a strong, supportive family who would be with me throughout the operation itself. This request caused a considerable conflict at home. Mom and Dad were both very busy, and they did not see the need to take four days out of their lives to sit around hospital waiting rooms while I got checked out. I expressed my concern about being difficult and antagonizing the transplant team. My parents said they should only have to come for a day to meet with whomever wanted to meet with them. I agreed, but felt that we should do everything the team wanted.

Dad called Ellen and asked if they could just come down on Wednesday. No problem, she replied. Once again, I felt like an idiot.

On a Sunday night, I checked into the hospital. The CF ward was in the Anderson Pavilion, a relatively new building in the hospital complex. The windows were small on the floor, which meant that most of the light came from fluorescence. This was muted by the warm, dark tan and brown hues of the walls and carpeting. I settled into my room and soon after I arrived, a nurse named Lucy came to speak with me. She outlined my schedule for the next three days. I would have an EKG and x-rays. They would do an echocardiogram on my heart. They would do a MUGA scan of my heart. The results of the MUGA would determine whether or not they would do a cardiac catheterization test on me. They would do a lung profusion scan of my lungs. I would do a six-minute walk test. I would be screened by the transplant team's social worker and psychologist. I would meet with the anesthesiologist. In other words, I would be busy.

Lucy said something else to me that stuck out because it was so unusual. She told me that a resident on the team named Dr. Mark Stang would be coming to see me and that I was lucky because he was very smart. Nurses don't usually provide unsolicited opinions about doctors.

I flipped on the Disney Channel, watched the animated version of Robin Hood, and began to relax. Then Dr. Stang came to see me. He was an inch or two taller than me, and had a very earnest expression. I peppered him with questions. A new anti-rejection drug called FK-506 was in the middle of clinical trials. Was the UNC team using it? They were looking into it. *The Wall Street Journal* had recently run an article about new techniques in asking for organs. It suggested waiting for the deceased person's family to accept their grief before asking for organ donation, not asking at the moment the person was declared brain dead. Would this affect the supply of organs? UNC was very good at organ procurement. At what point on the list would UNC ask a person to move down to Chapel Hill? Approximately three months before transplant, when they were number three or four on the list. What was the MUGA scan? It measured my heart pressures. What type of chest physiotherapy would I need to do after transplant? Minimal post-surgery, and then none. After transplant, sodium intake is restricted. CF patients get dehydrated very easily and are on a high sodium diet. How did that reconcile? I would not be as prone to dehydration after transplant. How long after transplant could I start lifting weights? After a few months. I would have to allow time for my sternum to heal.

Dr. Stang then gave me a checkup. He again went over my schedule and explained it to me. The heart scan and the lung scan both used radioactive dye, so they had to be conducted two days apart.

On Monday morning, a tech came to take my blood. She ended up taking seventeen tubes of it. Among other things, they ran a test for HIV. A positive reading would have disqualified me for transplant. They began a twenty-four hour urine collection. I met with the anesthesiologist, who explained my pain-control options. He advocated using an epidural, a small catheter inserted into my spine post-surgery. It would totally block the pain, he said.

Will Crowder, the team social worker, stopped by my room. We did not hit if off well. He told me that we were scheduled to meet Tuesday. He said that our meeting was very important and that I should be on time. He looked as if he spent the bulk of his time in crisis mode, putting out fires.

Then I went down to nuclear medicine for my MUGA scan. There a tech inserted an IV in my arm with amazing ease. He had me lay on a small, uncomfortable metal table. Then he maneuvered the scanner above my chest. He shot the dye into my arm, and the scan ensued. It did not take long, he yanked out the IV, and I was soon on my way. I then had an EKG which was normal.

After the EKG, I went to PFT's and blew an FEV1 of thirty-six percent. That meant that the amount of air I blew out in the first second of a forced exhalation was one-third that of a normal person. I never put too much stock in the actual numbers. They went up and down all the time, and hanging my hopes and fears on their vicissitudes would be emotionally draining. I knew if I felt good or bad. That was most important.

Next came the six-minute walk. It improved since my first one, to 2070 feet. This time, though, I didn't inflame anybody's bursitis.

For the last two hours of the afternoon, I met with the team Psychologist, Eileen Burker. With short, blonde hair, glasses, and an easy-going bookishness, she reminded me of Dr. Walden's intellectual sexuality. We hit it off right from the start and had a good conversation. I was fairly certain that I passed any psychological criteria she had.

I checked out of the hospital and into my old stomping grounds, the Hampton Inn. Then Rachel Burnett and I went out for Pizza on Franklin Street, the main drag of Chapel Hill. Her doctoral work was progressing well, and she was now dating a businessman up in Washington.

During the second day of my evaluation, I had a bone density scan. People with CF often get osteoporosis. It is not understood why. This test would determine how strong my bones were. They felt good and I was confident that like all of my other tests, I would sail through this one. The bone density test was difficult in that I had to lay on my back, perfectly still for almost an hour, as the scanner slowly inched up my body, shooting it in long cross-sectional shots. It studied my spine, hips and femur. I tried not to cough, but it was very hard.

After the test, Ellen stopped by to tell me that the results of my MUGA scan were in. With CF, because the lungs are constantly congested, the heart has to work especially hard. This can cause it to become enlarged. My heart, however, was healthy and I would not need the cardiac catheterization test. Hooray.

Will Crowder contacted me to change our appointment to Wednesday.

That night, Mom and Dad arrived in town and we went out to dinner at a pasta joint on Franklin Street. The place was packed and we would have had to wait an hour for a table. But a middle-aged couple invited us to join them at their table. This was typical behavior for North Carolinians: outgoing, friendly, and giving.

On Wednesday, I had the lung perfusion scan. Like the MUGA, a tech began an IV on me. I laid down on another uncomfortable table, and he placed a scanner above my chest. This time, however, I had to lay still for a while, longer than the time spent on the MUGA and shorter than the duration of the bone density scan. I tilted my head and could see the radioactive dye on the screen, slowly perfusing into my lungs. My right lung was twice as bad as my left lung, at a perfusion ratio of sixty-six percent on the left to thirty-four percent on the right. This meant that during my transplant, the surgeons would remove my right lung first. It also meant that if I got very sick in my left lung, my health could take a sharp turn for the worse.

After my lung perfusion, we were scheduled to meet with Ellen Cairns and Dr. Frank Detterbeck, a transplant surgeon. The team was in the middle of performing a transplant, and Ellen stepped out of the Operating Room long enough to tell us that she didn't have time to meet with my parents. That was totally fine with us. We wanted the current transplant to be a success. Dr. Detterbeck, however, would be able to meet us in an hour or so.

I had never met him before, but had heard good things about him. Apparently, he had a very social personality. We waited for him in the physical therapy department because I was now an outpatient and he had nowhere else to meet us. When he finally came around, he instantly reminded me of the actor Richard Dreyfuss. He had a mustache and the same warm but mischievous smile. Nobody else saw the similarity, but I'm sticking to it.

Dr. Detterbeck was Dr. Egan's back up. If Dr. Egan was out of town, or if they had to perform two transplants at once, Dr. Detterbeck filled in. People had whispered to me that Dr. Detterbeck was just as good as Dr. Egan. In the end, there was no way of knowing who would be performing

a particular transplant on a particular day. You just had to place an enormous amount of trust in the team. I had no problem with that.

Dr. Detterbeck told us that the transplant team met every Tuesday.
He explained that the team meeting included everyone: physical therapists, nutritionists, psychologist, social worker, transplant coordinators,
pulmonologists, and the surgeons. At the next meeting, they would
review the results of all of my tests and determine whether or not I
should go on the list.

Mom and Dad say that Dr. Detterbeck came off as very conservative
and cautious. He told them that transplant was "not a walk in the park."
It was high risk, the odds were only 50% survival at the five year mark,
and the procedure was relatively new. A successful transplant was not a
foregone conclusion. In essence, I would trade in one set of problems
for another.

This gave my parents "great pause."

After meeting with Dr. Detterbeck, we met with Will Crowder, the
social worker. That turned out to be a disaster. He had a spiel that he
had to recite to us, that took at least an hour. He asked if we could
afford the transplant. We assured him that we could, but he went on
to explain the costs in great detail. He said that the primary price
determinant was the amount of time a person had to spend in the
ICU after the operation. Some people healed slower than others and
had to spend a few weeks up there. That could double the cost, from
one hundred and fifty thousand dollars up to three hundred or more.
He said that he could help us fund-raise if we had to.

Then he began his routine about the importance of patient compliance. Right about then, my blood sugar crashed. I was very hungry and
it was well past my usual lunch time. I was tired from three days of testing, and he was questioning how well I took care of myself. It was an
absurdity to even waste time discussing it. If he wanted to know the
truth, he could call Dr. Chernick or Dr. Rosenstein, both of whom would
swear that I did a very good job. Will could have opened my chart and

seen how much I did above and beyond the call of duty. Or he could have just looked at me to see my good weight and strong muscles.

Will struck a nerve and I tried to maintain self-control as I answered him. Later, Mom and Dad told me that I totally blew a gasket. They had never seen me get angry like that before. They were convinced that at the team meeting next Tuesday, he would vote against me.

After we left our meeting with Will, he came rushing out and caught up with us in the courtyard just outside of the cafeteria. What did we plan to do about reconciling our religious beliefs with receiving a transplant? We had no clue what he was talking about. "Jehovah's Witnesses do not believe in blood transfusions, which are sometimes necessary during transplant," he said. We explained that we were Jewish and had no such qualms about blood transfusions. Apparently, the hospital computer coded me as a JEH instead of a JEW.

We ate lunch, and then headed back through the hospital towards the parking deck. In the main lobby, we bumped into Eileen Burker and Dr. Paradowski. Eileen spoke with Mom and Dad, while I spoke with Dr. Paradowski. It was only the second time I ever met Dr. Paradowski. I told her that I was about to go through hockey school. She surprised me by saying that she was a huge Buffalo Sabres fan. She told me to have fun playing.

CHAPTER 5

❀

The 28 Month Wait

I returned to Bethesda in the beginning of December. Within a week, hockey school began. Also, within a week, Ellen called to tell me that I could consider myself officially on the waiting list. Both were entirely separate events that seemingly had no relationship with each other. After all, being placed on the waiting list resulted from events that first unfolded a year earlier. I had waited for hockey school to start since May. But in retrospect, I think they converged on my life at the same time for a reason: self-definition.

Playing hockey enabled me to define myself in a very positive manner. It allowed me not to exist solely as a sick person waiting idly. It allowed me to express the tenacity that lurked inside. It allowed me to focus on something completely outside of myself. It was over-the-top and extreme.

After I registered and sent in my check, I learned a horrible fact about the sport: most amateur games are late at night. School took place at 10:45 p.m. in Reston, Virginia, twenty minutes from my house. It ended at 12:30. Ironically, the late hour proved beneficial for my respiratory therapy. It allowed me plenty of time to do my routine of nebulizer, Vest, and Flutter before leaving the house.

On my first day of school, I arrived at 9:45, not knowing a soul. Most of the people that showed up didn't know anyone else either. There were two teams that would be going through school together, the Heat and the Fanatics. I was on the Heat. We were given green practice jerseys and green socks, which, combined with our bright red helmets and pants, made quite an ensemble. We clamored into a locker room and gagged as we smelled the toxic, post-game sweat of the team that had just departed. After recovering, we began changing into our gear. Unfortunately, we had no idea how to put any of it on. Which did you put on first, the shin guards or the pants, the shoulder pads or the gloves? It was very confusing, but somehow we made it onto the ice.

Reston had two rinks, an enormous "Olympic" sized rink and a regular "NHL" sized rink. Our classes would be held on the Olympic ice. This meant that each lap was bigger, and each time we would skate down the ice as fast as possible, it was longer.

Our coaches worked us mercilessly. They had us warm up, skating a few laps. That in itself killed me. Everyone skated so fast that I could barely keep up. Then they had us stretch. We each had to stand against the boards, and raise one skate at a time up to the top, thereby stretching our hamstrings. I couldn't get my skate up that high, so a coach came over and yanked it up. By some miracle, he didn't rip the muscle.

After we loosened up, they began to teach us the basics of hockey skating. The hockey stop. The cross-over. Skating backwards. Skating forwards and turning around to skate backwards without stopping. Crossing-over backwards. They had us skate very fast and then dive onto the ice head-first. When we did so, we didn't feel any pain, and realized how well padded we were. "Everybody grab some ice" the coaches would yell. When they said that, it meant we had to lie face down on the ice to start a drill. I actually looked forward to those moments because it meant I could rest for a second.

By the end of that first lesson, I was exhausted to my very core. Sweat had run down my face, stinging my eyes, for the entire second hour. I had been afraid that I would freeze wearing only a thin jersey and pads in a cold rink so I had worn long-johns. Never again. That thin jersey and those pads were plenty warm. We got back to the locker room and I looked at the faces of my teammates. Many of them appeared as tired as I was.

It took me an entire week to recover from that practice. I could barely walk for a few days and my muscles felt sore right up until the following Thursday. This was not good. I pulled one of the coaches aside while we waited for the Zamboni to finish clearing the ice before we skated onto it. I asked him if our games would be a lot easier than hockey school. Because if it wasn't, I didn't see how I could cut it. He said that games were much harder because there was the motivation to win. But then he told me to stick with it, that things would get easier.

Sure enough, it only took six days for me to recover from our second practice. Then five. Then we had two weeks off for the Christmas holidays. Even though I worked out and skated on my own those two weeks, I lost the conditioning edge that I had built up, and paid a heavy price when classes resumed. It again took me seven days to recover after our first practice after break.

When I played, I coughed. The high impact aerobic aspect of the skating really shook up my mucous, and I would occasionally have to skate over to the players' bench and spit into a trash can. Sometimes there was no can back there which forced me to spit onto the concrete floor behind the plexiglass boards. The rest of my teammates seemed to spit directly onto the ice when they felt the need, but I couldn't do that because my mucous was thick and green, not thin and clear like theirs.

Skating that vigorously made me lose my breath. I would huff and puff after each drill, holding onto the side of the rink to keep my balance. I remember panting so hard that my diaphragm muscles heaved involuntarily, exchanging as much air as possible. I felt like the character Evinrude in the movie *The Rescuers*. He is a dragonfly who loses his breath every time he flies somewhere. He is so out of breath that his entire body is constantly wracked in convulsions.

Practice would end at 12:30 in the morning. By the time I changed and drove home, it was usually about 1:15 a.m. I would immediately gulp down lots of water and eat lots of pretzels to prevent dehydration. If I became dehydrated, the mucous in my lungs would become thicker and not drain properly, which could lead to serious infections. I would buy the pretzels that contained the highest salt content available, 800 mgs per serving. Then I would inhale an extra nebulizer bronchodilator treatment.

Hockey produced in me an incredible endorphin high. Combined with utter exhaustion, it created a strange buzz. I was wired, but calm. Even after showering, I was still totally pumped up. It would take me at least an hour to fall asleep after getting home. Slowly, my body began to acclimate to the sport. Slowly, my teammates got to know each other.

In February, we began to play actual games. We still weren't completely sure how to put our gear on, and we had absolutely no idea where to stand on the ice. When we started playing games though, I really began to enjoy the sport.

At first I played winger. On our second game, I had an assist. Even so, I did not have that scoring drive. After a few games, we found ourselves short a defenseman, and I volunteered. While I was not mentally attuned to scoring goals, I relished the ability to stop our opponents from doing so. I really loved defense, and have played it as much as possible since then. Defense was very similar to the role I played on Mrs. Fisher's soccer team as a kid. On the soccer team, I was a defensive halfback. I had joined the local soccer team in fourth grade. A number of my friends were on the team and encouraged me to sign up. My dad did as well: "They've got great uniforms," I recall him saying.

We were coached by Sue Fisher, our goalie's mother. She stood taller than most of my teammates' fathers, and bore the air of a highly organized and efficient individual. She was Martha Stewart with cleats. Mrs. Fisher always had the line-up planned out well in advance; the team balls were always clean and fully inflated; and the field was always crisply lined. During our games, her willowy frame would pace up and down the sideline as she clutched her clipboard close to her chest. She focused on the action more than most of the players. At one point or another, we all entertained precocious and inappropriate thoughts about her. She was a soccer mom long before the 1996 election made them a hot commodity.

Mrs. Fisher bore one unique quality that made a deep impact on me: she motivated us in a very positive manner. No matter which corner of the field we congregated at, and no matter how poorly we happened to be performing, we could hear her thin but confident voice: "Good job, Kenneth. Way to go, J.T." She never berated us. Not once. Sometimes, we would look over at the opposing sideline and bear witness to a coach screaming at a kid for a bad throw-in or a weak corner kick.

Hockey and soccer are similar enough that I could translate many of my instincts from one to the other. In April, hockey school ended and I was sorry that the season was over. I immediately signed up for summer league, but that wouldn't begin for two months. The thought of a hiatus tore me up. Then I got sick.

∗∗∗

I've often found that even though the doctors, antibiotics, and respiratory therapies are usually the same, there is something different to each hospitalization. There is no such thing as truly routine. Maybe it is because a disease is an ongoing process.

On this occasion, my routine deviated when I began to cough up a small amount of blood. This condition is called hemoptysis and is fairly common in CF. The repeated lung infections cause scarring in the small airways, and those scars can sometimes rip. I went to Baltimore and Dr. Rosenstein admitted me to the hospital.

If the hemoptysis is mild like mine was, IV antibiotics can clear it up. As soon as the bleeding started, I stopped doing my Pulmozyme, Flutter, and Vest, which can all aggravate it. If the bleeding is heavy, then doctors have to do a procedure called a pulmonary embolization. They insert a catheter into a vein in the groin and loop it up into the main pulmonary vein. They then proceed to the bleeding vein and block it off. This works but increases the pressure on the rest of the veins supplying the lungs, thereby making future episodes of hemoptysis more likely.

This admission was pivotal in two ways. First, I changed my mind about vegetarians. Being a card-carrying carnivore, I had always thought that I could never marry a vegetarian. But at Hopkins, I had the most beautiful physical therapist who happened to be of that persuasion, so I dropped the qualification.

The second pivot that took place concerned where I would receive my IVs. After five days in the hospital, Dr. Rosenstein came to my room and suggested that I could finish my course at home. My hemoptysis had cleared up quickly without the need for embolization and the IVs were working well. I would have better food, and could take very good care of myself. I was a bit nervous, but he told me that he had patients who were seven years old who had mastered home IVs.

Debbie Rownaghi, a former pharmacist at the CF Pharmacy, now worked at a home infusion company and I called her up. She explained the intricacies of home IV therapy to me. A nurse would come over and start an IV. It would be a little bigger than the ones I had previously, but would be more maintenance free. It would last for the duration of my therapy. Instead of being a one-inch plastic catheter, this would be six inches. That made me very nervous, but Debbie told me not to worry. The catheter would be inserted in a narrow form, then expand a little a few hours after it was inside my vein. There would be a nurse and a pharmacist on-call twenty-four hours if I had any problems.

I immediately took to home IVs. I could be with Bogart. I could sleep in my own bed. I had privacy. And I could eat food that hadn't sat on a plastic tray in a service elevator for an hour before being served.

✳✳✳

I finished my novel, *Target Market* in May, a year after I began writing it. Then I started sending it out to agents, editors, and publishers. Not a nibble. So I began rewriting it. We went up to Cape Cod in August.

Then, I injured my eye. I had been napping and woke up coughing very hard. I stood up quickly, still coughing, to get a Kleenex. When I stood up, I blacked out momentarily, and woke up on the way down. It was too late and I landed on my face. It didn't hurt but my eye began to fill with a little bit of blood. Over the next few days, more blood entered my eye and my doctor told me to have it checked out in the emergency room. The doctor told me that my vision was excellent. I could read two lines better than twenty/ twenty. But the blood would take a month to clear up. During that month, I got plenty of stares. One pudgy kid on line in front of me at a hockey rink gaped at me. I asked him if I looked scary. "No," he replied. "Just gross." I cracked up.

Once or twice in the past year, I had blacked out if I were standing up when I coughed hard. So if I started to cough, I made sure to sit down quickly. That was the extent of the problem. Ian Ferguson suffered much worse blackouts, and doctors had no idea what caused them. They were "idiopathic," which, he told me, meant that the doctor was an idiot and the patient was pathetic. Ian also began to have severe hemoptysis. This happened almost daily, even after completing a course of antibiotics. He went on the waiting list at UNC one month after I did.

✳✳✳

Early in September, I met Jane. She worked out at my gym. Jane had smooth brown hair that she pulled back behind her ears. Her ears drove me absolutely crazy with desire. She wore tight-fitting outfits and had a husky voice. She worked in human resource management, finding jobs for recent immigrants. On weekends, she worked with kids at a local gym. She lived with her mom and liked Asian food. I told her about my health right up front and she accepted it.

At first, we hung out together at a Watergate pool party. Then we went out on a date. I took her to the circus. Within a week, our relationship got intimate. We were inseparable, talking to each other many times a day, starting first thing in the morning and ending late at night. She called me all the time, as I did her. We were totally stupid and giddy together. I'm sure we were annoying to be around.

One day soon after we started dating, I had to see a new doctor for insurance purposes. After the basic exam, he began asking some personal questions. First he asked me if I had a girlfriend. I said I did. Then he asked me if I really loved someone, how could I ask them to assume all of my health problems? In essence he was saying that I had nothing to offer anyone. I thought of Ian and Suzanne and knew that while their health problems were significant, they were wonderful spouses who offered a great deal to Lindsay and Jim. I knew that the doctor was way out of line in saying what he said to me. Even though I had some self-confidence, it was very upsetting to be confronted about the issue by a total stranger.

As a lover, Jane had an unbelievable wild streak. She was creative, enthusiastic, and untiring. She had sexual preferences that I had never even thought of before. She initiated encounters in my car and in Rock Creek Park. I enjoyed it so much and I liked her so much, that I refused to jinx it by bragging to my friends. I admit that I was falling hard for her.

But after a few months, she started to act differently. She was less available to go out. She called less frequently. She had been asking a million questions about my transplant and I tried to be completely honest.

That candor probably scared her. I can understand that. Her father had passed away from cancer when she was only four years old, and she did not want to expose herself to that again.

One night, we planned to go out to dinner at Ruby Tuesday's, then to a hockey game of mine. I couldn't wait for her to see me play because I thought she might find it arousing. While we waited for a table, we went to a womens' clothing store next door. There, she modeled miniskirts to wear to work, asking how they looked. They were all very sexy, but not the best thing to wear to the office, I told her.

At dinner, she told me that we should still date, but should begin seeing other people as well. I disagreed. We were well past the point where that was appropriate. Why did she feel that way? I asked. She said that we didn't have enough in common. This was absurd. Like what? I asked. "You bought a shirt at J.C. Penny," she replied. "I could never buy anything there." Actually, it was a very sporty shirt and I always received compliments when I wore it.

Jane went on to say that my health was a major deal breaker for her. This was the first time anyone had come right out and said it to my face. She came to my game that night in Reston, and I was so mad that I pounded the hell out of the other team. The next day I told her that I didn't want to hang around the sidelines of her life. It sucked and I was devastated.

I couldn't understand why a person who had very strong feelings for me did not have the character to fully accept my problems. Ian Ferguson had married a wonderful woman, Lindsay. Suzanne Pattee married a great guy, Jim Tomlinson. Many people I knew with CF found spouses that looked beyond the health issue. But Jane could not.

Chapter 6

Rising up the List

Nancy Schlossberg, a friend of the family, joked that in the beginning of 1996, our family had to shut down for repairs. I got very sick around Christmas time. I had almost enough hemoptysis to merit an embolization, coughing up a cup of blood over a few days. I had a bad lung infection. I was resting at home one day and Karen rented the Jim Carrey movie, *Dumb and Dumber*. One particularly hilarious scene involved a scatological disaster with Jeff Daniels. It made me laugh so hard that it put me over the top. I went into the bathroom and coughed up a good bit of blood into the sink. It spattered onto the wallpaper and onto the floor, and it took me a half an hour to scrub it clean enough so that nobody could tell. For the following week, every time I went in there, I noticed tiny specks of blood, camouflaged by the wallpaper.

I began home IVs, and they started to work, but slower this time. The bacteria that colonized in my lungs began to develop resistance to the antibiotics. The first time I used IVs, back in high school, I felt a significant improvement within a few days. This time it took over a week to get that effect.

Early on in my course of IVs, a terrible blizzard came through Washington, dumping three feet of snow on the region. The roads were virtually impassable, and the plows were not even attempting to clear back streets like ours. My home IV company had to bring me a new supply of medicine and check my blood. Somehow, they got within a few blocks of my house in a sport utility vehicle. Then an extremely dedicated nurse, Suzanne Vazzano, hiked in the rest of the way hauling my medicine.

Home IV technology had made a big leap. Now, each dose of my medicine was contained in a balloon the size of my palm. The balloon was protected by a hard plastic shell. The system was designed to squeeze the medicine out at a predetermined flow rate, such as 150 ccs per hour, controlled solely by the elasticity of the rubber. There was no need for a cumbersome pole or pump. The balloon could be placed in my pocket and I could roam about as I pleased.

It could even work while I did my nebulizer and my vest. For the past year or so, if I got sick, I would bump up my routine from three times a day to four times a day. This meant over six hours of chest pt. It was consuming, but effective.

The blizzard was rough on Bogart. The snow was deeper than he was and I'm sure he held it in for two days straight rather than get a little wet. I was too sick to go outside and shovel a clearing for him. The poor guy began to look green, not easy for a black dog. After a week, the snow began to melt, and the roads began to clear off.

One night, Grandma came over for Chinese takeout with my mom and me. After dinner, we played a rousing game of Scrabble. Grandma was a champ and had taught me how to play when I was in elementary school. Unfortunately, she liked to develop a few of her own rules to the game. At one point during our match, I made the mistake of disputing one such rule. She got very mad, and went on to beat the heck out of us.

Four days later, she went into cardiac arrest and died. Mom rushed her over to nearby Suburban Hospital, but they could not save her. I wished I could go over there to be with Mom, but I couldn't. I was stuck at home in the middle of an infusion. I was also scared of going into a new hospital and exposing myself to all of the germs that floated about.

Grandma went quickly, but it was still very hard for us. Cousin Jonathan and his wife Ruthie flew in from Chicago. Although he was not a rabbi, he conducted the funeral service. Jonathan's parents, Lenore and Michael, flew in from Dallas to offer their support.

***

Getting *Target Market* published turned out to be quite a challenge so I reworked the novel. Soon after I finished that draft, the company that manufactured the ThAirapy Vest came out with a new model. Instead of weighing one hundred and ten pounds, it now weighed thirty-five. That was a machine I could travel with much more easily. As I waited to hear from the agent, I became very superstitious. Each morning, I would check my horoscope first thing. Oddly enough, a significant number of days referred to publication and advertising. It was bizarre. I treated fortune cookies with great care. I would save the best ones and scotch tape them to my computer. At one point, I saw an infomercial for the "Psychic Friends Network" and seriously debated calling them to see if they had any insight into my getting published.

In May, I traveled back to UNC for clinic. That morning, I went to physical therapy so that they could pound on my chest. The tech who usually worked with me was not available so someone else filled in. She would play an important role in my transplant. Annie Downs was a full-fledged physical therapist. It was clear that she had done chest PT for years and years. She knew just how to cup her hands to get the right sound, and she knew how to keep a good rhythm going. With chest PT, there are many different positions that can be done and patients get to

know which positions work the best. After a while, they begin to focus
solely on those. Annie was very thorough and encouraged me to go
through all of the positions. One of the first things I noticed about
Annie was that she wore a very appealing perfume. It was spicy, like
Opium, but subtler. As she pounded on my chest, I scooted slightly
closer to her on the table to smell it. Annie had a compact body, all muscle. She had strong facial bones that resembled a Comanche chief's, perfect skin the color of creme caramel and super white teeth. She
maintained a very relaxed but alert expression. She didn't miss a thing.

After PT, I proceeded on to clinic. Dr. Aris told me that I was still too
healthy for a transplant, and that I should come back in six months. If
I rose too high on the list, meaning that I could be called if a good
match became available, they would make me inactive. The time that I
had accrued would still count to the Carolina Organ Procurement
Organization, and when I did need new lungs, I could go active again
with all of that time behind me.

Dr. Aris also told me that my Epstein-Barr antibodies had not yet
converted. The Epstein-Barr virus is a serious risk after transplant. The
virus itself can cause mononucleosis and chronic infections. It is linked
to numerous types of cancer and chronic fatigue syndrome. For transplant patients who do not have the antibodies before the operation but
then obtain them from their donor, the risk of lymphoma in the first
year post transplant increases significantly.

The antibodies for Epstein-Barr are common to most people. Dr.
Aris suggested that I go out and kiss lots of people to try to gain those
antibodies. This would enable me to convert prior to transplant.

As I left clinic, I bumped into Dr. Egan. I asked him a question about
the mechanics of the operation. With his finger, he traced the incision
across my chest, from one armpit to the other. It gave me goose bumps.

After returning to Maryland, I joined a mystery writer group, "Sisters in Crime." SinC focused mostly on assisting female authors. It held monthly luncheons and had interesting speakers.

I started attending those SinC lunches in the summer of 1996. The group consisted of mainly female mystery writers and readers. They were mostly in their forties and up, and had a real passion for mystery in all of its permutations. They had police dog and firearms demonstrations; speakers talked to us about forensics and fraud. It was fascinating and I loved each event that I attended.

***

That summer, I began to swim regularly. My parents had built a pool in the backyard a few years earlier, but I rarely swam in it. I liked the water very warm, and nobody else liked it that way. This is my one neurosis: I play ice-hockey, but hate water cooler than eighty-four degrees. Usually, by mid-summer, a few heat waves would naturally jack the water temperature up to the mid-eighties, and then I would be very comfortable.

I eventually realized that swimming helped me sleep better. When the water got warm enough, I went in and swam a few laps. That night, I did not cough as much as on other nights. There were far fewer Kleenex by the side of the bed in the morning. I tried swimming again and the results were the same. Now, I had to swim to get a decent night's sleep. But the water soon cooled off. So I went out and bought a wetsuit. There, in July, in Bethesda, I would don the wetsuit and comfortably swim laps. Everyone except Bogart and my friend Jan Lastuvka thought I was completely insane.

Jan and I had first me in Junior high and had become friends in High School. He began life within the iron curtain and only escaped because his mother carried him across the Czech border as an infant. He has since risen to become a very successful engineer.

There are a few reasons why swimming helped me so much. First, the aerobic nature of the exercise forced open my small airways much like using the Flutter. Another reason is that at the surface of the water, the air is perfectly moist. This makes the activity a combination of exercise and nebulizing.

***

On August third of that year, I got a phone call in the early afternoon. My friend, Ian Ferguson's sister, left a message on my answering machine: "Ian's got new lungs. He got out of surgery at 12:30 and he's doing great." He had gotten the call Friday night and flown down from Maryland with his wife, Lindsay. He felt that he didn't have too much longer. He was having massive hemoptysis on a daily basis, and needed IVs often. He had looked very haggard and thin for a while. I sent him a card that expressed how I felt: "I'm so happy for you that my smile muscles hurt."

Ian had been another patient of Dr. Chernick, and I had met him at NIH in 1987. He wore free-spirited skateboarding t-shirts and surfer shorts but his unwavering eyes and short crew cut revealed an internal sense of military discipline. He studied architecture at Catholic University. The day that I met him, he had just gotten dehydrated working at a construction site in the Washington heat. Our relationship became one of dual mentorship. From my end, I taught him how to take better care of himself. He began coming with me to the gym at the local Jewish Community Center to lift weights, and he began receiving chest PT from my physical therapist. He took to weightlifting immediately, reading up on the sport and educating himself far beyond what I taught him. Ian's mentorship of me would evolve after his transplant.

The very night of Ian's transplant, Amy Goldberg got married. She had met Chuck Kines two years before and had known immediately that they were meant for each other. She had told me that she met someone, and that he was very, very, short. When I met him, he was exactly my height, and I've given her a hard time about that ever since. Chuck came to our *Melrose Place* evening one night, and expressed the feeling that the show was not his cup of tea. He wanted to take a pass on it in the future. But soon, he started coming every Monday, and that's when I knew it could be serious. .

Chuck listens to the Grateful Dead and has a "Peace" bumper sticker on his car. He does not eat meat. He is an avid outdoorsman. His bachelor party consisted of white water rafting in West Virginia.

At their wedding, I went around and told everyone who would listen about Ian's transplant. I was so happy. I danced with a number of beautiful women. I pigged out on the buffet. My friend Jon Hefter utilized his "buffet stacking system," enabling him to heap about three layers of food onto one plate. This is why the two of us get along so well.

A few days after Ian's transplant, I called Jean Rae, the new transplant coordinator, to see how he was doing. Ellen's husband had been transferred to Germany so she had to leave UNC. Jean told me that Ian was doing well. He was out of the ICU and up and about.

Then she shocked the hell out of me. She told me that I was now number two on the list. It was time for me to get a beeper. I had last been to UNC for clinic in May. At that time, Dr. Aris told me that I was still too healthy for a transplant. My health had not changed at all since May, so I didn't understand why my status should. I was still playing hockey. I asked her to review that decision carefully. I even offered to come down there even though I was not scheduled for another visit until October. That was not necessary. The doctors reviewed my case, and concurred that I should get a beeper. Jean also told me that they would ask me to move to North Carolina when I became number one on the list.

Will Crowder, the social worker who I had such problems with initially, stepped up to the plate. He helped me coordinate the beeper. And he helped me coordinate air travel. I would need to have a charter air service on standby so that if organs became available, I could be down in Chapel Hill within two hours. UNC had a backup Air Ambulance on standby that could come up and get me, but that would take longer. Will also told me that I should start attending transplant support group in Chapel Hill. There I would learn much more about the operation.

The beeper companies provided beepers for free to patients awaiting transplant. It would not display a phone number when it went off. It would only tell me that someone was trying to page me. In other words, I could only give the beeper number to one person: the transplant coordinator in Chapel Hill. There had been problems of abuse by other patients and the beeper company was trying to protect itself. That was fine with me.

A week after receiving my beeper, I drove over to Amy and Chuck's for *Melrose Place*. Halfway there, my beeper went off. I freaked out. I rushed to the nearest pay phone and dialed the hospital operator at UNC. She paged the coordinator on-call, who happened to be Kristi Gott. Kristi had been in charge of patients post-op. Ellen, and now Jean, had been in charge of patients pre-op. Kristi told me that she was not trying to reach me. False alarm.

I ended up having four false alarms in the ensuing weeks. Each time, I would pull off the highway to find the nearest pay phone. They had told me that if my beeper went off, I had fifteen minutes to contact them. Kristi and I got to know each other well. Finally, I called the pager company and begged for a model that showed phone numbers. That way I could recognize a false alarm without going into a full panic. They agreed.

As soon as I got the beeper, I started calling around charter air services in the Washington area. There was one run out of a small airstrip in Gaithersburg, Maryland, that, for a thousand dollars, could fly me and my parents down to Chapel Hill. They could be ready within an hour, long enough to find a pilot, and they could have me there in an hour and fifteen minutes. They promised to be on standby for me, and asked that I check in regularly with them to keep apprized of my status.

***

In mid-September, Dad and I flew down for our first support group. It was a warm, sunny, fall day in Carolina, and it felt good to be back. Every other Wednesday, Will held a support group for people waiting for a lung transplant. The purpose was to educate those waiting so that they knew what to expect when their time came.

Ian was the guest speaker that night. He was six-weeks post transplant, and he looked terrific. It was the most-rested I had seen him in years. The dark sacks that had hung below his eyes had disappeared. I picked him up at his rented apartment, and he showed me all of his medicine. He showed me a notebook he had that explained each drug and had a schedule of when he was to take them. He also unbuttoned his shirt and showed me his scar. He now mentored me.

Because they had flown down in the middle of the night, Lindsay had rented a completely furnished apartment. It was in a brand new development, a cluster of four-story apartment buildings. Theirs was on the first floor so that Ian wouldn't have to struggle up any stairs. It was very spacious. And it had a view in back of the woods. Along with the furniture, they had rented pots and pans, sheets and towels. Their two-year-old daughter Ashley had come down soon after the operation, and the cyclone of her toys gave the place a very homey feel.

Lindsay's employer, Oracle, had been incredibly supportive. She had taken some personal time off, and then worked out of their apartment in Chapel Hill, tele-commuting. They would live down there for three months after his operation, until November. That was standard protocol.

Support group was held in the clubhouse of another apartment complex. The facility held a pool, from which we could smell the chlorine. There were also two squash courts, which provided the constant sound of hard rubber balls pinging off the walls. I looked around at the other patients and realized that I was the only person waiting who was not on oxygen.

***

The transplant team added a third coordinator to their group: Judy McSweeney. Judy had worked as a nurse in the pediatric intensive care unit for five years, until Dr. Egan recruited her. This was her first support group and Will introduced her to us. She sat on a barstool with her hands stuffed under her legs and her heels resting on a bracket. She had a warm grin and a sense of openness. It was clear that she was eager to learn. Her tan face was bathed in the glow of love for her new job. Judy's neck muscles were incredibly well defined. Like booster rockets abutting her windpipe, they firmly supported a delicate face and hinted at high-caliber athleticism. She looked very conservative in a white summer sweater and long pants.

Judy and I had spoken on the phone a week earlier. Our first conversation concerned swimming. She asked what I had been doing that day and I told her I just came home from swimming. I had switched pool venues for the Fall, from our home to the JCC, which miraculously kept its water at eighty four degrees. Judy asked how far I went. I didn't want to answer, but she coaxed it out of me. Three laps up and back. She mentioned that she swam as well. How far did she usually go? With reluctance, she finally admitted: "two miles, in open ocean."

Because of the rising number of patients, the team had reorganized its coordinators. Instead of having two coordinators, one dedicated to pre and one to post, now three people split the patient load and followed one person before and after. I had been assigned to Judy's caseload.

After support group ended, I went over to speak with her.

She and I struck up a casual conversation and were soon joined by Mary Ellen Smith, another person waiting. Mary Ellen was in her mid-forties, weighed one hundred and seventy pounds on a five-foot four body, and had an oxygen cannula running from her nose to a portable tank. She had a very jovial manner. Mary Ellen had a disease called Kartangners. That caused the cilia in her lungs to be damaged or missing. She had been born with her internal organs reversed. Everything that was supposed to be on the right side was on the left, and vice versa.

Judy asked us how our illnesses affected us. Mary Ellen answered immediately. "Honey, it just means that Gerald has to be on top." With that she rocked her ample pelvis back and forth as if to demonstrate. I burst out laughing and Judy turned a bright red. I knew Mary Ellen and I would be instant friends. "You are a wild woman," I told her.

After support group ended, Dad and I went out to dinner with Ian. He had gotten to know the restaurants of Chapel Hill and suggested a popular place called Crook's Corner at the far end of Franklin Street. It was best known for its shrimp and grits, and had a large pig on the roof. The three of us were shown to a table in an enclosed courtyard filled with quirky sculptures and began to sit down. I noticed ash trays on the table and people smoking nearby. I immediately asked the hostess to move us to non-smoking. Inhaling smoke would immediately make my small airways constrict so I avoided it. Ian told me that not only would he not have noticed any smokers, but that they would not have bothered him. That was an incredible change. Two months earlier, he would have been less able to tolerate smoke than me. Then I noticed his appetite. He could always eat a hearty meal, but now, he put me to shame. First he started with a massive plate of hush puppy appetizers. Then a generous salad. Then a huge steak and fries. Finally, he tossed back some pie and ice cream. It was wonderful to behold. Ian told me that transplant would make my appetite explode. Dr. Egan told people not to buy any new clothes right after transplant because they would soon outgrow them.

Two weeks later, Dad and I came down for another support group. This one was lead by Jean Rae. She explained all about pain control options after transplant. She advocated the use of the epidural, but said that sometimes, doctors couldn't use it for various reasons. One such situation was if a person had to be placed on blood thinners during the operation. She said that after a few days, we would be given a hand-held PCA, or patient-controlled analgesia. This would be a button that we could press that would give us morphine as we needed it. If we felt that we needed more than the PCA allowed us to have, doctors could change the settings to allow that to happen. The team's whole approach was to make sure we were comfortable. That way we could breathe easier and start walking sooner, two important components to recovery. She underscored the point that we should expect some discomfort, but we should let them know if we were in pain.

In mid-October, Dr. Egan gave his annual talk at support group. The Ramsgate clubhouse was standing room only. Annette and Jay came, as did Ian and Lindsay.

With his usual blunt humor, Dr. Egan explained the nuts and bolts of the operation. He brought along slides and made it look easy, not unlike the way Michael Jordan makes a tomahawk slam dunk look easy. There were three basic connections that had to be made in a lung transplant: the pulmonary artery, the pulmonary vein, and the main airway. First they would make a "clamshell incision," from one armpit to the other. They would saw across the sternum but not through any ribs. Then, they would pop the patient open like the hood of a car, raising the entire ribcage to gain access to the lungs. The surgical table would actually bend in half to make that easier. Then surgeons would take out the worse lung, put in a healthy one, and repeat the procedure with the second lung. It would take eight to ten hours.

Dr. Egan described the differences between single and double lung transplants. For CF, he had to do a double lung transplant because otherwise, the bacteria from the old lung would migrate into our new lung and infect it. Most of the patients in the program had CF, but about twenty-five percent did not.

Dr. Egan spoke about the shortage of organs, and what that meant for us. He told us how many people died waiting each year. He explained that lungs were difficult to retrieve because other organs like the kidneys had to be removed first. He said that lungs had a unique advantage in that they stayed viable much longer than other organs, for up to twelve hours.

Then he told us about research in transplantation. People were studying xenotransplanation, or animal donors. He felt the most hopeful research looked into ways gunshot victims and heart attack victims could become donors. He said that if their organs could be used, that would virtually eliminate the entire two year wait.

After he spoke, Dad and I walked over and had a conversation with him. Two nights before our trip down, the TV news-show *48 Hours* ran a story about patients who wake up from anesthesia during major surgery. The condition is called "awareness" and is very rare. Doctors know that the patients were awake because they later can accurately recall the conversation in the OR. My friend Tom Faraday, who had his transplant in Pittsburgh, told me that he woke up during his operation. His eyes were still closed, and he felt no pain. But he could hear what was going on. So he concentrated all of his attention on wiggling his big toe. The doctors saw that and put him back under.

After watching *48 Hours*, I was concerned about awareness. I asked Dr. Egan if that were a risk. He told me that it had happened to him once, and the patient was able to tell him what was said during his surgery. But Dr. Egan went on to explain that sound is the lightest sense. When we wake up in the morning, it is usually from hearing a noise rather than from experiencing light or touch. That's why a person can wake up just enough to hear something but not feel it during surgery before they put you back to sleep. This seemed to assuage my fear and I didn't think about it anymore.

I met Charity Fennel, who had received a transplant and heart repair one month after Ian. Charity came from Florida and had been extremely sick prior to her transplant. She had bright red hair like Pinky Tuscadero from Happy Days, cropped very short. Like Ian, she wore a surgical mask inside the support group to avoid exposure to CF patients with lung infections. She was now immuno-compromised and had to be careful.

Then Judy pulled me aside. She told me that it was time for me to move down. I had become number one on the list. I wasn't sure what chain of events occurred to bump me up, but I again asked if they were sure. She said that they could recheck my records, but I should make plans to move down.

I didn't sleep for more than an hour that night. I lay awake in my room at the Hampton Inn, thinking about transplant. After flipping channels for three hours, I determined that there was absolutely nothing on television. There was nothing to read in my room besides the "Welcome to Chapel Hill" guide and the hotel's safety instructions. Dad had the car keys in his room so I couldn't go out and drive around, and I did not want to wake him. So I lay awake and stared at the walls. I worried that I might still be too healthy for the procedure. Dr. Egan had told me that I was far better off with my own lungs, and I did not want to make a huge mistake that could potentially shorten my life. The winter hockey season had just started and I felt terrific. I had not done any IVs since my grandmother died.

In the end, I decided that if lungs became available and I was not ready, I could always pass on them. But not being sure as to whether or not I was ready, I wanted to position myself to receive them in the best way possible.

CHAPTER 7

Number One

Mom, Dad and I debated whether or not I should move to Chapel Hill. My parents felt that moving was unnecessary. After all, Ian didn't have to move, so why should I? I knew that Ian's circumstances were different than mine. His wife had a full-time job that she could not leave. He did not want to be separated from her, and the transplant team understood that. Ian flew down when he got beeped. Michael Boyd, another patient of Dr. Chernick's, received new lungs at UNC a year before Ian, and he too, did not have to move to Chapel Hill because of his wife's job. Michael actually drove to Chapel Hill from Maryland when he got beeped.

I felt that with winter approaching, storms could hit that would make travel difficult. What if my lungs came during a severe winter storm and I could not make it down to North Carolina? That would be a terrible reason to miss them. Even though Ian got beeped in the summertime, he almost missed his lungs because most of the area's pilots were away at a convention.

I felt that the transplant team knew best. If they wanted me to move to Chapel Hill, I could meet that request.

A week later, Mom and Dad flew down to Chapel Hill for the weekend to hunt for apartments. After numerous endeavors over the years, I am convinced that apartment hunting is one of my dad's many splinter skills. They found me a great place within an hour. I was set to move down to Chapel Hill on November 14, 1996, one week away.

Before I left, Amy and Chuck hosted a "new-lung shower" for me in their new apartment. Amy made a huge poster of a stork delivering lungs. She bought a huge medical poster of the complete respiratory system. And she hung streamers all over the place. They invited about fifteen people over for a great sendoff. My *Melrose Place* crowd pitched in and bought me a pizza stone and a pizza paddle. Mike Simpson bought me a pack of cigarettes "since you don't need your old lungs anymore."

It was difficult to say goodbye to my friends. It was also difficult to say goodbye to my hockey teammates. We were five games into the Winter season. As I played my last game with them, I wondered how long it would be before I played hockey again. That made me sad, but I threw everything I had into that game to make the most of it.

As I prepared to move, I made two purchases. First, I bought a winter jacket. My old one was shot, and I wanted to buy a ski jacket in a cold climate like Maryland. The other purchase I made was a pair of running shoes. I knew that much of my existence in Carolina would be dedicated to working out on treadmills and stairmasters, and I wanted to be prepared.

My last stop before I left was my dog Bogart's vet, Dr. Benson. In 1988, my parents gave me the dog for my birthday, a black standard poodle. I am convinced that his personality has to be the result of his birth near the Seabrook nuclear power plant in Rye, New Hampshire.

Bogart had severe socialization problems. He could not handle being around other dogs. He hated squirrels, motorcycles, UPS trucks, and just about anything else that stimulated his overactive chase reflex. He loved eating trash, and kept a running mental inventory of our waste-baskets. He ate anything he could dig his teeth into, including metal, plastic, wood, and the TV remote. It did not surprise anyone when he developed colitis.

The vet attributed Bo's problems to lots of nervous energy and suggested that I had to run him every morning. So I began bringing him to doggie play group at the park. This took a slight edge off of his behavioral problems, but he still needed obedience school. I took him to three separate trainers. He flunked each and every class. The first one may have been my fault because I was more interested in Laurie, the trainer, than in actually teaching the dog how to heel.

Now in November of 1996, Bogart was still very neurotic and would bark at the slightest provocation. I feared that if he acted up in my new apartment, we might get thrown out. He was about fifty pounds over the legal limit there, and I didn't want to rock the boat. So I asked the vet for Prozac. I had read that they now prescribed it for dogs and I thought that it might be a good way to take the edge off. The vet refused, saying that it would not help him.

✳✳✳

The day before I was set to leave, Ian called and said that he needed to head down to UNC to see the doctors. Did I want some company for the ride down? Heck yeah.

We crammed my computer, clothes, and some pots and pans into the car, carved out some room for Bogart in the back seat, and headed South. That entire trip, we talked about transplant. He shared with me all of his experiences with totally honesty. His biggest fear before his transplant was the bronchoscopy. For the first year after transplant, doctors conduct the procedure at regular intervals to make sure that there is no rejection or infection in the lungs. The "bronch" is a long, flexible tube that they insert in a nostril and guide down into the lungs.

With it they can take tissue samples, or biopsies, and visually inspect the airways. Ian said that his fear turned out to be unfounded. They doped him up so well that he usually slept through it.

I shared with Ian my biggest fear: the urinary catheter. That was pretty much my only concern. Ian assured me that when it was in, you couldn't feel it. They inserted it while you were still asleep, and the only time you felt it was when they yanked it out. And that he felt for only a second. Even so, I was not convinced. I was afraid that they would take it out before my system was ready to start urinating on its own, thereby forcing them to put it in again. That happened to Tom Faraday numerous times. He said that it didn't bother him too much, but I refused to believe him.

Ian told me about the medicine in greater detail. At about two o'clock in the afternoon, just after we crossed over the North Carolina border from Virginia, his hands started shaking. He told me that it was caused by Cyclosporin, and usually happened as the level of the drug peaked in his system. He opened up a small cooler that he had brought along and drank a bottle of orange juice. Soon his hands stopped shaking. He said he was getting used to the shakes.

Ian explained to me what life was like being immuno-compromised. Because of the risk of the body's rejecting the new organs as an outside invader, transplant recipients take drugs to lower their immune system. This exposes them to greater risk of contracting infections. Ian was on his way to North Carolina to have one such infection examined. He took the whole thing in stride. "Whatever the problem is," he told me, "they can treat it." He had complete faith in the transplant team.

We arrived in Chapel Hill at my new development, Summit Hill, late in the afternoon. The buildings were all two tones of gray with white trim. Gentle roads curved through the complex. There were pine trees and weeping willows, and a huge lake with a fountain. There were tennis courts, a pool, and a hot tub. This would be a very easy adjustment.

The apartment looked very nice. It had three bedrooms so that Mom, Dad and Karen could all converge on Chapel Hill at the same time. With windows on three sides, the apartment was very sunny. There was a balcony with French doors that overlooked the woods. And it was on the first floor at Ian's suggestion. The rented furniture was all in place.

I soon discovered one drawback to Summit Hill. It was situated next to the Farrington Road Waste Water Treatment Facility. The sewage treatment plant was well hidden behind the woods, and nobody mentioned its existence to my parents. Soon after I moved in, however, a strong odor rolled over the small hill that separated my building from the facility. It smelled like stagnant sea water fermenting with seaweed and clamshells. That didn't bother me. Once a month, though, a truly fetid stench would settle over my building and the parking lot.

Aside from that, Summit Hill was terrific.

Soon after unpacking, I picked up Ian and we went out to dinner at his favorite Chinese restaurant. It was conveniently located about two miles from my apartment. Unfortunately, I did not share his appreciation for the place. That would be my only real gripe with North Carolina: I could not find decent Asian food anywhere. It wasn't long before repeated disappointments led me to give up the search and focus on foods that the area prided itself on, like barbecue.

That night, I locked the door to my apartment and smiled at Bogart. We had our own place once again.

✳✳✳

The next morning, I had transplant clinic. It was Friday. I arrived at ten and met with Dr. Stang. He listened to my chest, and then asked me a question: "Why do you think you need a transplant?" I explained how I spent five hours a day on chest pt; my infections seemed to be more frequent; if I got a cold now, it would inevitably lead to a lung infection; if I got a lung infection, it would most likely involve hemoptysis.

Dr. Stang leaned back in his plastic chair, and declared: "That's not enough. You're too healthy." This the day after I picked up and moved down, a fact that he was well aware of. Judy McSweeney stood next to him and I could see that she was furious that he made that comment. She held her tongue and asked him to go outside to confer. I told him that I wanted them to be damn sure that the time was right for me before they did a transplant. He agreed, and said that if they did a transplant too soon and it did more harm than good, it would be a terrible thing. He said it with a tremendous amount of compassion. It struck me as unusual for someone so young to understand that concept so well.

He stepped outside with Judy and then returned with Dr. Paradowski. If they did me that day, I would be the healthiest person in the program's history to get new lungs. That would be a good thing because I would recover very quickly. I would probably set a record for getting out of the hospital, she told me. Dr. Paradowski said that I should go get a set of PFTs. If my FEV1 fell below thirty percent, I should stay on the list. That was fine with me.

Before I headed upstairs to the PFT lab, I spoke briefly with Kristi Gott. She reiterated the importance of being in good physical condition prior to transplant. She had one patient, Chris, who went skiing two weeks before his operation.

As I rode the elevator up to PFTs, I worried about how on Earth I would tell Mom and Dad that a day after moving down here, the team decided I wasn't ready. That would be a huge emotional drain on all of us. It was very upsetting for me.

I arrived at PFTs and recognized the technician, Gary, from my evaluation two years earlier. I told him the stakes that were involved in this set of numbers. He was very laid back and just encouraged me to blow hard. My first two blows registered twenty-nine percent. My third blow hit thirty. Over the years, I had taken so many PFT tests that I knew how to maximize every blow. There were a few secrets to cheating on them. Don't eat anything for two hours prior. Make sure your bowels are empty. Hold your breath for two seconds before the forced exhalation. I knew that I was not at optimal PFT condition. I was tired from moving down the day before and my blows would not be as strong as if my lungs were rested.

By this point in my life, just taking PFTs could be a challenge. Doctors liked there to be three blows that had similar numbers. Sometimes, however, the numbers varied greatly, and the techs would make me blow over and over and over, until either we got three equivalent results, or I was too exhausted to go on. Attaining three similar blows was an unrealistic expectation. The exhaustion of repeated trials would make the numbers go lower and lower, and the initial results were far better than the ones at the end. Ian told me that sometimes he would take as many as 16 different tests in one sitting.

Looking strictly at the numbers that day, I did hit thirty percent. Even so, Dr. Paradowski felt that I should be on the list. I trusted her.

Ian got very sick that weekend. I called him to check and see how he was doing. The doctors had admitted him to the hospital and were going to operate on him Saturday afternoon. They had found a sac of fluid behind his heart. He was in a really bad mood because nobody told him what was happening. He didn't mind the thought of surgery. He did mind the lack of information he was given.

✷✷✷

My first weekend in North Carolina, Annette, Jay and I went out. They made me feel so welcome. First we had pizza in my apartment. Then we went out to the movies. We saw *Swingers*, an independent film that had a profound impact on me. It was about a cool guy who teaches a less suave friend how to score with women. Annette declared that I was the dorky guy in the movie. I am convinced that watching the movie helped my social life in North Carolina. From that point on, I dated more women than I did in Maryland. After I watched it, I called all of my single guy friends back in Maryland and begged them to go see it.

That weekend, I went through serious hockey withdrawal. The thought of not playing for a long and indefinite period of time made me depressed. Kristi's words in clinic skittered back and forth across my conscience. "Chris had skied two weeks before his transplant." If he could ski, why the heck couldn't I play hockey? Then I opened the Raleigh News and Observer and saw an ad for an adult hockey league. I called up and they described their league as being very similar to what I played in at home: no fighting, no checking, and they had a "C" level for people who were not too good. I picked up the phone and called Mom. "Can you send me my hockey gear?" Sixty dollars and three days later, a UPS truck pulled up and dumped it all on my doorstep.

It turned out that Ian had a small, infected sac of fluid behind his heart. Instead of opening him up completely to remove it, doctors drained it and he recovered quickly.

The following Monday, I reported to pulmonary rehab in the physical therapy department. Annie Downs ran the program. Rehab was scheduled to begin at 2:30 in the afternoon. This was very inconvenient because normally, I was napping at that hour. I would have to do all of my nebulizing, Vest and Flutter immediately after lunch, walk the dog, and rush right over to PT. If I wanted to nap, it would have to be afterwards. If I napped beforehand, I would miss my respiratory therapy. Rehab began at 2:30 because the rest of the day was booked up. The entire morning was dedicated to patients post transplant. They worked out in two shifts. The one o'clock time slot was assigned to Brian Urbanek. He had undergone a transplant three years earlier, but because of rejection, had to go on the list again for a second transplant. He had to be kept separated from the other patients waiting because he had a strain of bacteria that was resistant to antibiotics. It had colonized in his lungs. That left the two-thirty slot.

Before I started, I had one big fear about rehab. Would it cut into my weight lifting and swimming? After all, I could only workout so much per week. If I had to spend three days on a treadmill and stairmaster, would I be too tired to do the types of exercises that really paid off? I had one other concern that completely contradicted that fear. The stairmaster was very difficult and I had never been able to last for more than four minutes on it. How would I hold up?

When I arrived, there were two other patients getting ready to work out. One was a young woman named Melissa Ogden. I couldn't tell her age. Either she was a teenager, or a young adult. I recognized her because she had been sitting directly in front of me during Dr. Egan's speech. The other patient was Brett Pearce. He was a senior at UNC. They both nodded at me, but neither spoke. After seeing *Swingers*, I was now in "Mr. Cool" mode, so I nodded back.

Annie explained the set-up to me. I would work out on two machines, one for thirty minutes, the other for twenty. As she spoke, Brett climbed on a Stairmaster and started working out. Melissa began on a treadmill. They also had stationary bikes. I could pick whichever machines I wanted. They would monitor my pulse-ox throughout.

A tech strode over to a mini-rack stereo system and asked what we wanted to listen to. She then popped in a "No Doubt" CD. From that point on, she was our deejay.

Annie took my blood pressure and weight, and asked where I wanted to begin. I suggested that I start on the treadmill. It was hard. For five minutes, I warmed up. Then Annie raised the grade slightly and sped up the machine. For the next twenty minutes, I huffed and puffed. I watched Melissa on the next machine over completely whip my butt. Brett was cranking away on the Stairmaster, sweat dripping off his face. He now had an oxygen cannula looped under his nose because his oxygen saturation had dropped below ninety percent. Even dependent on oxygen, he was going hard for thirty full minutes, twenty-six longer than I could have done. It didn't take long before Brett and Melissa started insulting each other. Brett directed blonde jokes at her, and she returned fire. If they were not yet dating, I thought they should be. For the last five minutes of my treadmill workout, Annie dropped the grade back down to zero and the speed back to my warm-up rate.

Finally, I was done, and I rested. The tech offered me a cup of water.

Then Annie asked what I wanted to do for my second machine? I let her decide. How about the Stairmaster? Sure.

My first time out, I lasted eight minutes. That was double the length of time I expected to last. Halfway through, however, my oxygen saturation dropped to eighty-nine percent and Annie put me on oxygen.

While I rested afterwards, I asked Annie where I could find a pool. She suggested a few health clubs and the YMCA. When I got home that night, I opened up the phone book and started calling them. "What temperature do you keep the water at?" The Chapel Hill "Y" was the warmest at eighty-four degrees.

✳

I'm not sure where I first met Michael Ackerman. It was either in clinic, support group, or rehab. He was waiting for a double lung transplant and lived in Winston-Salem, about an hour and a half away. He attended support group and rehab once a month. He was thirty-seven, tall, and wore broad brimmed, straw golf hats. He looked very serious. He was dependent on oxygen all of the time.

We spoke occasionally and became friends. His interests were varied and he was a Jack-of-all-trades. It turned out, he was a very talented artist. He also worked as an apprentice book binder and as a television producer. A devout Christian, God played a prominent role in his life.

CHAPTER 8

❀

Adjusting to Life in North Carolina

After rehab that Monday, I opened up the Yellow Pages and started calling around for a cleaning service. I needed somebody to help clean up once a week. After unpacking, the place already needed a good scrubbing. The first number I called belonged to "In-house Cleaning Service." I left a message and a woman named Sherry Williams called back. She wanted to take a look at my apartment before giving an estimate.

Sherry came over at seven. She was a very substantial woman. When she entered a room, she owned it. She could win over anyone. Even Bogart, whose sociopathic tendencies seemed to surface when he met a stranger, offered her his tennis ball. She threw it for him, and they became friends. A pair of sunglasses rested on top of her head. We got to talking and she gave me a good estimate. She could start with her crew that very week. We could coordinate times so that it wouldn't interfere with pulmonary rehab. Sherry told me that on weekends, she was a Baptist minister. When I told her about my transplant, she took a genuine interest. She promised to pray for me. Sherry started cleaning my apartment once a week with her crew.

I went to rehab on Wednesday and found that my endurance was rising. I could do a steeper grade on the treadmill at a faster speed, and I was able to climb twelve flights on the Stairmaster. On Thursday, I joined the YMCA. The Y was located near Chapel Hill's tiny airport, about fifteen minutes from my apartment. Like the Hampton Inn, pine trees surrounded the building and shaded the parking lot. I didn't know how soon my transplant would take place, which meant that I didn't know how long I should join for: one month, three months, or six months. Judy felt certain that my transplant would occur before the New Year, but it was really anyone's guess.

So I joined for one month. I went downstairs to the locker rooms, changed into my swimsuit and showered. I took my gym bag with a box of Kleenex out to the pool and was struck by the view. One entire wall consisted of floor to ceiling glass windows that faced out into the woods. I could see a small pond visible down a gentle hill. It was idyllic. The water was very warm and I got in easily. As in Maryland, I could only swim three laps.

***

Bogart adjusted well to North Carolina, although at first I worried about him. Every time I returned home to my apartment, I noticed him staring out the window to the parking lot. The poor guy missed me. Soon I realized how wrong I was. Even when I was at home, he spent all of his time looking out that window, his considerable snout resting on the low sill. He had become the neighborhood busy-body, constantly monitoring the comings and goings of each person that lived in our end of Summit Hill.

Bogart liked the nature in Carolina. Behind our building lay a huge meadow. Sometimes if we went walking back there early enough, we would see deer. The first time he spotted them about one hundred yards away, he gave me the look of a curious hedonist discovering opium for the first time. He practically said: "what are those and how can I get one?"

***

Thanksgiving rolled around and Mom, Dad, and Karen drove down to visit. On the way, they realized that they forgot to bring a set of sheets for my parents' bed, so they had to hunt for it. Every store was closed for the holiday. Finally, in South Hill, a strip of gas stations and fast food restaurants an hour north of Chapel Hill, they found a Rose's Department store that was open and sold linen. Mom could not understand the saleslady's thick accent. To her it sounded like an uninterrupted, high-pitched string of vowels. She has imitated it ever since.

I cooked a big Thanksgiving dinner for everyone, which was ready when they arrived. Being so new to town, I had forgotten to buy Paprika, which made browning the bird a bit of a challenge. I managed with a little cinnamon.

The next day, my high school class had its ten-year reunion back in Bethesda. Our five-year had been a great bash. This time I could not attend. At eleven that night, I got a call from the reunion. Seventy-five drunken people all got on the phone to wish me well. By this point in the evening, many of them had impaired language skills so their exact words were a little muffled and slurred. Their spirit, however, came across loud and clear and meant so much to me.

That weekend, Mom and Karen found many small things wrong with the apartment, things I had never noticed. The oven didn't heat properly. The shower pressure was anemic. The water went cold halfway through filling the tub up in the master bathroom. Through her constant telephone calls to them, Mom became good friends with the handymen for Summit Hill, Beau and Bill. They kept coming over and fixing each problem.

Aside from the small inconveniences, my family liked North Carolina. Dad brought his golf clubs down and we hit a few buckets of balls at a driving range nearby. Karen liked the men in Carolina and their accents. As soon as she arrived in the state, she began listening to country music. I began to suspect that she might write her doctoral dissertation on lyrics specific to that genre. Mom seemed to be making friends everywhere she went: from Duke and UNC to the Southern Seasons gourmet food store. When she and Dad were at the furniture rental store getting me set up before I moved down, the stress in our situation must have shown on their faces. A very large woman worked her way over to Mom and said: "Honey, you look like you need a hug." Strangers were friendly and warm, a far cry from Washington D.C., and Boston.

It was sad to see my family leave at the end of our Thanksgiving weekend, but my life in Carolina was starting to pick up.

The following week, I began playing hockey in North Carolina. My new team, the Pirates, played about once a week over in Raleigh. Usually games were on a Monday or a Tuesday night. Depending on which it was, I adjusted my pulmonary rehab schedule accordingly. I couldn't do rehab the day after hockey, so if I had a Tuesday night game, I skipped rehab on Wednesday. Annie gave me permission.

My teammates on the Pirates had been playing for a few more years than me and were much better. They came from all walks of life: Robert worked for the Postal Service. Mike was a CAT-scan technician at Duke Medical Center. Mark was a television newsman. They welcomed me to the team and, like the Heat back home, they totally accepted my health.

There were a few differences between my old team and my new one. In Carolina, there were far fewer players, so most games we played short-handed. Because hockey is such a grueling sport, a person plays for shifts of one or two minutes, then rests. Normally, there are three people who share each position on the ice. Everyone plays one-third of the game. Since there are five positions besides the goalie, you need fifteen people to field three lines. With ten people, you can field two complete lines. Our team in Maryland usually played with between ten and fifteen people, so we always had at least two lines. In Carolina, we seemed to play many games with seven to eight guys. This meant that there was very little time to rest. My teammates, though, let me rest as long as I wanted.

The one drawback to my Carolina team was that I wasn't good enough to play defense, the position I loved the most. After one game at "D," Robert asked me to play forward. I agreed, but wasn't happy about it. Then I started to get into the groove at forward, and didn't mind it.

When I started playing hockey in Carolina, I felt like a character in the Tom Clancy movie *The Hunt For Red October.* In the movie, a Soviet submarine commander defects to America. He evacuates his crew and makes them think he is single-handedly battling the American Navy. The sub's doctor declares with great pride: "The Captain is fighting them." By playing hockey, I felt as if I too, were fighting.

By now, my workout schedule for the week consisted of pulmonary rehab twice, hockey once, swimming once and weightlifting once or twice. I found myself exercising six days a week, my resting day being the recovery day after hockey. The swimming, hockey, and weightlifting were all carried over from Maryland. Pulmonary Rehab was the only new ingredient to the mix. The improvements I noticed in my endurance, therefore, must be credited to it. After a few weeks, I could swim four laps instead of three. Twelve flights on the Stairmaster had grown to twenty, then forty. It was paying off.

At rehab, Brett, Melissa, Brian and I were getting to know each other. There was some healthy competition between us to see how well we could do on the machines. Brett usually killed us. He would raise the treadmill to a twelve percent grade and crank the speed up to four miles an hour. I had progressed to an eight percent grade at 3.5 miles an hour. Melissa worked out at about my level. Once a month, the therapists conducted six-minute walk tests on us. Brett usually could do about 3,300 feet. When I started, I did 2,088. Soon after rehab began, that number started to rise. After a month, I was up to 2,600 feet. A month later, I got up to 3,200. I was so proud that I e-mailed all of my friends about it. The next day, Melissa beat me on her test by 100 feet and I was crushed.

Brett was the president of UNC's *Star Wars* club. He studied pre-med and English lit. He was applying to medical school. His sister Kim had undergone a transplant three years prior. Another sister, Kim's twin, had died of CF a few years earlier. To this day, I am amazed at how hard Brett worked. He was extremely motivated to graduate on time and go to med school. When he had to go to the hospital for IV antibiotics, he would go out on pass to attend class. He pulled all-nighters to get papers done. And he earned stupendous grades. For fun, he would pile into a car with his friends and road trip down to Florida to root for UNC in the Gator Bowl.

Melissa came from Oklahoma. Her mother, Angie, moved with her and they stayed with her grandmother who lived forty-five minutes away in Fuquay-Varina. She loved Arby's roast beef sandwiches. She had a one hundred and fifty pound bull-mastiff dog back home, a pet that probably weighed a third more than her.

Melissa's health became a problem for her before she had the opportunity to go out in the world and enjoy life as an adult. She had graduated from high school but had not yet been able to go to college.

Although Brian worked out before our group, we got to know him during the changing of the guard. He was very well educated. He read a great deal, enjoyed dance and art, and had lived in New York City before moving to Carolina. Professionally, he had worked in marketing for Xerox.

In December, I contacted the Tarheel Chapter of Sisters in Crime. By coincidence, North Carolina's group met in Chapel Hill. I had a long conversation with the chapter president. Her brother awaited a kidney transplant. She invited me to the group's potluck Christmas dinner. I whipped up a batch of quesadillas and brought them.

I also remained in contact with the Chesapeake Chapter back home. Just before I left, their newsletter announced that Sisters in Crime pocket calendars would be on sale at the December luncheon. I wanted to buy one, but had already moved to Carolina. So I called the head of merchandising, Marji Hankins and explained to her the situation. No problem, she said. She would mail me a calendar and when I got it, I could send her a check. In the middle of December, I received my calendar, along with a card. The entire chapter had signed it at the luncheon and wished me well. The calendar was their gift. I had only just met them the previous summer, yet they acted in such kindness. I immediately taped the card to the wall in my kitchen and showed off the new calendar to everyone.

Two narrow edges of my transplant world became delineated for me soon after my move. Two patients in the transplant program died my first month in Carolina. Both had CF. Mike Hatcher came to rehab once every other week. I met him there as we rode the stationary bikes together. He was from nearby Cary, North Carolina, and worked out close to home the rest of the time. In early December, he got new lungs. He progressed quickly, leaving the Intensive Care Unit within twelve hours. But then he got an infection that he could not beat. He showed that transplant was not a cure-all for everyone.

I also met Angie Taylor at rehab. She was very sick and awaited a transplant. She was an in-patient. At first, she could barely get on the treadmill. Then slowly, we could see her strength progressing. Her stamina rose and she began walking with confidence. Like Mike, she didn't make it. She highlighted the importance of getting a transplant before my health deteriorated.

The following week, Mom and Karen accompanied me to support group. Will told us about their deaths. Most of us already knew. Will suggested that we take a moment of silence on their behalf. Then he said we could talk about it or not talk about it. "It's up to y'all." One person asked if they had done anything wrong to hasten their deaths. Did they fail to take their medicine properly? Will said that their deaths were not at all their fault. They did everything they could. Some people were very upset. Mary Ellen read a sad poem that she had written. Then I spoke up. I said that I had lost many friends to CF and when they died, it always made me work that much harder at staying healthy. In my own way, that's how I grieved for them. Maybe that's what we should take from Mike and Angie.

Karen came down to visit for the Christmas holiday. She quickly slipped into the Carolina lifestyle. Together, we found a wonderful, all-you-can-eat cafeteria in Raleigh. For seven bucks, we pigged out on some very good chow. We went and saw the re-release of *Star Wars*. I remembered when Dad took me to see it when it came out the first time back in 1977.

Karen came with me to rehab and got to know Annie. Annie gave us a transplant orientation. Angie Workman, a new therapist, also sat in on the session. Annie had a slide show that went through the process of rehab post transplant. It would start in the ICU. There, therapists would get me up and walking as soon as possible. She explained all of the tubes that I would have coming out of me. There would be four chest tubes to drain excess fluid from my new lungs and prevent my lungs from collapsing; a naso-gastric tube would prevent me from aspirating (vomiting and then choking on it); a urinary catheter; an arterial IV to measure my blood pressure and blood gases; a central line IV catheter in my neck; EKG monitors; and a pulse-ox on my finger. The therapist would load up the chest tube drainage boxes, called Pleur-evacs, onto a wheel chair which I would push as I walked. Annie showed us slides of people walking in the ICU, loaded with IVs and pushing the wheelchair that held their Pleur-evacs. Soon I would be moved out of the ICU to the fourth floor in Anderson Pavilion. As soon as my chest tubes were yanked out, I could resume rehab down in the physical therapy department.

Then Annie took us up to the ICU so that we could see what it was like and meet the nurses up there. Our first stop was the stainless steel sink. Annie explained that after the operation, people were immuno-compromised. As a result, they were very susceptible to infections. Family members had to be vigilant about washing their hands before visits. It looked similar to the ICU I spent the night in except that instead of the beige and orange paint on the walls, this ICU utilized a Tarheel Blue color scheme. There were a number of bays that held some very sick people. The lights were dimmed in most of the bays so that the patients could sleep easier. Each bed had a number of monitors above it, quietly blipping and beeping. For such a hard-core place, the nurses seemed very serene and in control.

After that orientation, I started mentally preparing myself through positive visualization. This was a skill that I learned playing hockey. Before every game, I would concentrate on all the things I wanted to accomplish during the game. Strong skating; moving opponents out from in front of my goal; keeping my stick on the ice. I would imagine myself doing all of those things. As I prepared for my transplant, I thought about healing quickly. I imagined myself waking up in the ICU after the operation. I thought hard about getting out of bed and walk-ing as soon as possible. I pictured myself pushing the wheelchair with the Pleur-evacs and doing laps around the ICU. If Mike Hatcher could be out of the ICU in twelve hours, I could too. When my time came to wake up in the ICU, I would be pre-programmed to move my rear.

During that holiday, Jon Hefter came down to visit. We had met in third grade but didn't become close until our sophomore year of high school. We both loved the writer Ken Follett, and we both loved busi-ness. In fact, Jon aspired to own a seat on the New York Stock Exchange. He is an expert windsurfer and a reckless skier.

We differ in that Jon always maintained a very neat demeanor. I remember his mother's concern before we went off to college that he wouldn't fit in because he was too much of a neatnick. My mom did not harbor a similar concern about me.

Jon is dyslexic and learning disabled. His teachers failed to diagnose him until his senior year of high school. Not only did he miss out on the bulk of his primary and secondary education, but he had to endure a lifetime of intellectual derision. To counter that cruelty, he cloaked himself in shyness.

When Jon visited me in Chapel Hill, he had just completed the first semester of his MBA at George Washington. By now, he had totally overcome his learning disability. Prior to attending graduate school, he had worked for an investment firm, managing four billion dollars in options. Now he excelled in school and developed self-confidence. It was great to watch.

Like Karen, he immediately took to Carolina. I felt obligated to point out every beautiful woman in the Triangle. While he and Karen were in town, I hauled out my new pizza stone. We learned two things very quickly: it was messy as hell and tasted very good. Our first mistake was trying to make a pie that was bigger in diameter than the width of the pizza paddle. We could not transfer the pie from the counter onto the stone. That pie ended up being rolled up into a stromboli. Our second mistake was being too liberal with the cornmeal. Cornmeal is sprinkled on the stone, the paddle, and the counter surface to make transferring the dough easy. We ended up with an entire kitchen coated in the stuff. Somehow it got into drawers that were never opened. It coated our clothes. And it dusted the floor.

A week later, I spoke to Judy about our experience. Like me, she loved pizza and owned her own pizza stone. She made a few suggestions, and listed her favorite toppings: spinach, artichoke and feta cheese.

***

The first woman I dated in Carolina was Juliette. She was finishing her Ph.D. in psychology. She had an artsy streak, drawing and making rugs. She had a sexy voice: clear, flirtatious, and confident. She drew out her words in long syllables, steeped in her New York accent. Her hair was wild, huge and explosive. It zinged out in all directions, untamed.

Soon, Sherry, who cleaned my house, set me up with Cathy. Cathy and I spoke on the phone and got along very well. She worked in anesthesiology research at Duke. She had lived on a ranch in Venezuela where she studied rare birds. She had gone to Yale and earned a degree in environmental biology. She spoke some Spanish and played ultimate Frisbee. She was very smart and interesting.

Then there was Amy. She had gone to my elementary school, junior high, and high school, and graduated two years after me. She just graduated from Medical School and was doing her residency at UNC hospital. Amy was a former athlete. In high school and college, she competed at a very high level. She played volleyball, softball, and basketball. Like Brooke Shields, she had thick eyebrows and a strong jaw. Even though she had grown up to be a striking, refined woman, she still looked like she did when she was in kindergarten. But now she wore earrings, drank wine, and saved peoples' lives.

CHAPTER 9

❀

A Major Setback

A number of people went far out of their way to keep me connected to the world. Mike Taylor called me on the phone from Maryland at least twice a week. He would tell me about the cases he worked on and life in general back home. Jon Hefter was now studying for his MBA. He called regularly to ask advice about the marketing projects he worked on in school. Every Monday night at nine, I would talk with my Melrose Place crowd and discuss important aspects of that week's show.

E-mail became a much larger part of my life. Like GIs away from home, I looked forward to receiving notes. A colleague of my mom, Warren Greenberg, made it a point to e-mail me everyday. Warren taught health economics at GW. We had some very spirited debates about the death penalty, Israeli politics, healthcare, and the Democratic Party. Through e-mail, I stayed in touch with Aaron in Texas, Karen in Boston, Mike Simpson in Maryland, and cousin Jonathan in Chicago.

Amy's husband Chuck e-mailed me a quote that I found very comforting. It was from *Random Acts of Kindness* and read as follows:

"When we come to the edge
Of all the light we have
And we must take a step into
The darkness of the unknown,
We must believe one of two things;
Either we will find something
Firm to stand on
Or we will be taught to fly."

I made a photocopy of the quote and gave it to Judy.

In the Army, troops in basic training have to scale a fifteen foot wall. I took part in a leadership conference during high school and we had to complete a confidence course that included such a wall. The secret to climbing the wall is that the group members pull each other up. People who make it to the top reach back down to hoist up others. With transplant, people who climb the wall pull others up as well. The mentorship I got from Ian, Tom Faraday, and Kim Brown about transplant continued with Laura Ferris. She and I had interned together at the CF Foundation years ago. Suzanne Tomlinson (formerly Suzanne Pattee) put us in touch. Laura now lived in Colorado. She had undergone a transplant a year earlier and she sent me an e-mail about her experience. She told me that ten months after her operation, she was "on her honeymoon, jet skiing in Barbados." That was a lot to look forward to. Laura told me that it took her six weeks before she felt like the operation was worth it, and she hasn't looked back since.

***

Midway through January, I got sick again. It wasn't a lung infection per se. I just coughed enough at night so that in the morning, I had thirty dirty Kleenex by the side of my bed. My lungs simply had too much mucous plugging my small airways. So I went to the CF clinic at

UNC. The Clinic was held in a new out patient facility, the Ambulatory Care Center, or ACC. It was a three story red brick building, modern in design and light and airy inside. It was located on the grounds of the hospital, but detached from it and a quarter of a mile away from the main buildings.

At the ACC, I met with a pulmonary resident, Dr. Sood and the attending physician, Dr. Rivera. Dr. Sood took care of me. I explained my situation and she felt that I should start a course of home IVs. She arranged the logistics with the home health company. She would be leaving the country in a few days, but she gave me a number to call if I had any problems. She did not expect any.

I bumped up my respiratory therapy regimen to four times a day; continued with pulmonary rehab; and because I had an IV catheter in my arm, I put hockey on hold for two weeks. I hired a neighbor, Craig Randall, to help me walk Bogart. Craig was in his first year at UNC law school. He had played football in college and was strong enough that I knew Bogart couldn't push him around.

After a few days, I had company. J.T. was in town on business with his partner, Sandy. I invited them over for dinner as long as they shopped for it and helped cook. They are both superb cooks, so I knew I was in good hands. It was great to see them, and it afforded me the opportunity to fill Sandy in on some embarrassing stories from J.T.'s wild past. There were plenty.

One afternoon, I went to rehab, which ended at about four thirty. I went back to my apartment but was too tired to cook. Then I realized that I lost my appetite and felt a little nauseous. Loss of appetite in itself is extraordinarily odd for me. I could not remember the last time that had happened. Maybe if I had a really good sub, that would inspire me to eat. So I drove into downtown Chapel Hill and looked for a sub shop. I bought a BLT and went home. The next morning, I called the number to the clinic and spoke with a nurse. She looked up the drugs I was on in a book and said that my symptoms were completely normal.

After a few days, I started to feel worse. Some minor hemoptysis started, which was unusual for the end of a two week course of IVs. My lungs should have been in good shape by then. So I went back to the CF clinic the next day, Friday. Dr. Sood was now out of the country, so I met with two new doctors, a resident named Dr. Tilley, and the co-director of critical care medicine, Dr. Jim Yankaskis.

Dr. Tilley looked just like Jon Hefter. He had the same long face, dark brown hair, and moppish forelock. He also shared Jon's shy bearing. Dr. Tilley asked what dose of antibiotics I was on. When I told him, his eyes popped out. It was double what the correct dose should have been. I had no idea. Two other doctors had checked the levels of Gentamicin in my blood and lowered the dose twice, both times leaving it higher than it should have been.

Dr. Yankaskis had a pale face, blond hair, and a thin body. He had a theory about the hemoptysis problem. IV antibiotics that weakened one strain of bacteria in my lungs might have enabled another strain to grow stronger. The delicate balance of microbiology in CF lungs can often shift when the bugs fail to keep each other in check. Dr. Yankaskis prescribed a new course of IVs with Vancomycin, a powerful drug that I had taken years earlier. They took some blood and sent me home.

Saturday, Mom and Dad came down to visit. We were scheduled to go out to dinner with an old friend. Early in the evening, just before dinner, I got very nauseous so I decided to stay in. Soon, though, I felt even worse, so I called the emergency number to the clinic. They paged Dr. Tilley. He offered to prescribe an anti-nausea drug for me. He said that he would be going into work Sunday morning and would check the results of my blood work.

Then he practiced superior medicine. He acted on an instinct and called the blood lab directly at nine that night. My numbers were completely out of whack. He called me ten minutes later and asked me to go straight to the emergency room. He would meet me there. My creatinine was 3.7. Normal was about 1.0. Creatinine is a protein made by the muscles. The kidneys clean it from the blood when they work properly. When they don't work properly, Creatinine builds up to dangerous levels. The IV antibiotics that I took were so toxic that they could cause renal failure. This is what he feared.

I had to wait for a few hours in the emergency room waiting room. After about two hours, Mom and Dad arrived. They looked around the waiting room at the mix of drunken college students and poor people with hacking coughs. They were afraid that someone might be contagious. They raised a stink and soon I was taken to a room.

There, two young interns began taking care of me. My lungs sounded good. The IVs had cleared the congestion of my small airways. They began cranking me with IV fluid.

The next day, Dr. Richard Boucher came in to take care of me. He worked mainly as a CF researcher, and was taking this month as his one month of the year to do clinical work. I had heard him speak at a CF Foundation board meeting a number of years earlier. Then about a week before I started using IVs, I recognized him in the local Harris-Teeter supermarket. We stood next to each other on the checkout line. I introduced myself and told him how much I enjoyed his speech back in Washington.

When he began taking care of me, he explained what may have happened. The Gentamicin was double the dose it should have been. It probably caused acute renal failure. He asked the kidney doctors to come and examine me. They agreed that it was best to monitor my Creatinine and BUN, another indicator of kidney failure. Dr. Boucher told my parents that I should be fine and that they could go back to Maryland. They were scheduled to go to Jamaica on vacation on Wednesday, and Dr. Boucher did not think they should cancel the trip. The next day my Creatinine rose to seven. The day after that, eleven. Dr. Boucher spoke with my parents and they came right back down. They would not be going to Jamaica. Karen flew down from Boston. They all looked very scared. Sherry, my housekeeper, took Bogart to stay at her house so that my family did not have to worry about him.

My body was completely poisoned and I felt unrelenting nausea. The nurses gave me shots of Phenergan which put me to sleep. That was the only time I felt relief. I was uncomfortable lying down, standing up, and sitting. Most of the time, I just sat on the edge of a chair with my head resting in my arms, which lay on my bed. I had raised the bed to its highest position. I could barely walk. In fact, I remember looking out the door of my room and being fascinated at how the nurses and doctors seemed to be able to move so easily. I went into the bathroom and for the first time, needed to hold onto the metal safety rail next to the toilet.

The doctors watched my urine output closely. I was urinating very little, two hundred ccs a day. Even that took great effort. I would imagine gushing bursts of water, Niagara Falls. The kidney doctors recommended a urinary catheter, but I refused.

On Tuesday, the kidney doctors determined that I needed dialysis. It would clean my blood by seven percent, but ninety-three percent would still be dirty. They would place a large catheter, a vas-cath, directly into a large vein in my neck. That made me very nervous, but by this point, I felt so bad that I wanted them to do anything to get me better. I felt like an ox to whom a heavy yoke had just been attached and was now required to pull a massive load.

I also felt a deepening sense that I was sub-human. I was not a self-sustaining unit. I could not be dropped in a forest and survive. I depended on medicine. I depended on other people. It was hard to admit. All I could focus on was fighting to get better.

The vas-cath insertion would be done by vascular radiology under a fluoroscope, which would enable the doctors to see my veins clearly. As I got prepped for the procedure, I got very nervous. I asked the tech for something to help me relax, and she said "No problem." The doctors there firmly believed that patients should be comfortable. Another tech came to administer some Demerol. He noticed that I wore my ice hockey jersey, and told me that he too played. Then I got stoned for the first time. Having the catheter inserted was relatively painless. All I felt was the bee sting sensation of the lidocaine.

An hour later, nurses hooked me up to dialysis. The first day was for a short period of time, an hour and a half. I slept through it entirely. Wednesday, I was alert throughout. It lasted two and a half hours. I brought magazines and the New York Times crossword puzzle. I never read them, though. I could not concentrate. Judy returned from a ski trip to Utah and visited me in dialysis. She brought me her own personal Walkman and some tapes. She had an incredible tan, but she looked very troubled about my health. She had sent me a postcard from Park City which I had taped up to the wall in my kitchen before I got sick.

The dialysis lab was a sad place. The other patients had been coming for a long time and were the walking wounded. A few of them were completely out of it. They would lie there and moan for hours on end as the machines scrubbed their blood. At one point, I saw one of the most disturbing things I have ever seen in a hospital. The nurses mimicked one elderly woman in a vegetative state. Witnessing that made me sick. It shattered the assumption that if you are out of it, people would respect you.

My family had a very difficult time seeing me in dialysis. The other patients looked so bad that it must have been hard for them to associate me in any way with them. And they were terrified about my health. I never could concentrate hard enough to share that concern. All I wanted was to get better. I still couldn't eat food, and didn't feel well enough to do chest pt. If I started coughing, I would vomit. During that time, I did the bare minimum amount of nebulizing possible. Since I could barely walk, rehab was out of the question. That negligence was hard, but I knew my lungs would have to take some slack for my kidneys.

Aaron called up from Texas to offer me one of his kidneys. The doctors never said that I needed a kidney transplant, but I felt really moved by his generosity.

The following Saturday, my family up and went to synagogue. That scared me. They never went to regular services. Now they were praying hard and I knew they must have some justification.

I worried about my status on the waiting list. Kidneys are vital to transplant. Kidney failure means automatic disqualification from being considered. I asked Judy and Dr. Paradowski if I should still wear my beeper. They said I could, but that I was temporarily off the waiting list until I got better. So I stopped wearing it. All I wore was my red Heat jersey and sweat pants.

Finally, after a week on dialysis, my kidneys recovered. My Creatinine began to descend back to normal. I began urinating again. Dr. Boucher told me to expect a deluge at first. When kidneys recovered, they worked overtime. He was right. For a few days in a row, I urinated eight liters a day. I was so happy, I told everyone who would listen. During this stage of kidney recovery, it is almost impossible to take in enough fluids to counter that excretion. Dehydration becomes a real danger.

I was discharged from the hospital and for a week, I lived solely on Gatorade. I still did not have an appetite. For a total of four weeks, I ate virtually no food. During that time period, I lost twenty pounds. I lost my sense of balance and constantly knocked against the walls. My eyesight was also affected. Images were not stable. They wobbled and blurred. Dr. Chernick said that I had probably been a few days away from going into a uremic coma.

***

The entire experience was completely avoidable. After I recovered, our family debated the merits of a lawsuit. A number of lawyer friends told us that we had a hell of a case. There were at least three major screw-ups involved. The doctor prescribed the wrong dose of antibiotics. The home health pharmacist failed to catch that mistake. The doctor did not confirm the dose with the pharmacist, as is standard policy. Twice, the doctors who lowered my Gentamicin dose failed to lower it to a safe dose. And none of the home health or clinic nurses caught the mistake.

We decided against a lawsuit for a number of reasons. First of all, my kidneys recovered and we were incredibly grateful. Secondly, we had fought so hard for so many years to raise money for CF research, we feared that a big settlement might somehow take money away from the research labs. Finally, we were still waiting for new lungs at UNC. We couldn't sue Sonny Corleone and date Michael. Like two of the Godfather's sons, one arm of the hospital worked with the other and if we sued one, we would be suing the other. I did not want to jeopardize my standing with the transplant team in any way.

If my kidneys had not recovered, that would have changed the situation. I would have not been allowed back on the transplant list. The immuno-suppressant drugs prescribed post-transplant are so toxic that the body needs to be able to filter them out properly.

Mike Taylor told me that I could sue the doctor personally, not the hospital. That was true, but I still felt that the transplant team might be affected. If I had died, my family most likely would have sued in a big way.

Dr. Paradowski told me that the one good thing about the incident was that I demonstrated incredible healing power.

CHAPTER 10

❈

The Final Stretch

A week after getting home from the hospital, Judy called to tell me there was a new problem. My blood sugar was out of whack and they had been following it for the past week. A reading of seventy to one hundred and twenty was normal. Mine was four hundred and fifty. I was really upset. To counter the risk of dehydration, I had been living almost exclusively on Gatorade. It was no wonder my glucose was high. Why didn't they raise the issue sooner? I could have changed my diet.

Judy suggested that I try diet Gatorade and eat salt bagels. My mom looked all over the area for it but could not find it. I suggested that she call the company. The company told her that they did not manufacture a diet version of their drink.

Judy wanted me to begin watching my blood glucose. She gave me a monitoring kit for home, so that I could check my own blood twice a day. That was incredibly difficult. We sat at a conference table in the hospital and she wanted me to stab myself with a lancet. I simply could not do it. Finally, she had me use a pen device that had a lancet auto-loaded. All I had to do was place the pen against my finger and press a button. That was a little easier, but still difficult. I hated it, but eventually, got a little used to it. Not much, though. My sugars dropped immediately after I stopped drinking Gatorade, but were still elevated. Dr. Paradowski prescribed an oral drug, Glipizide, which helped my pancreas produce the right amount of insulin. That did the trick. My glucose went back to normal. Dr. Chernick told me that the kidney failure was such a shock to my endocrine system that it made me diabetic.

A month after my kidneys failed, I went back on the waiting list. I feared that new lungs would come in for me before the rest of my body recovered. I had just started eating solid food again and I had to put twenty pounds of muscle back on.

As soon as I started eating again, I returned to exercise. I wasn't sure what to do first: weight lifting or swimming. Swimming would be aerobic as well as muscle building, so I went with that. I swam twice my first week back, combined with pulmonary rehab. There was a change at rehab during the month I was off. Angie Workman now ran the program. She grew up on a dairy farm in a small town in Iowa. She was my age, but seemed more mature. She was pregnant, laid back, and like Annie, a very good therapist. I soon discovered that she was a big devotee of disco music. She brought in her disco tapes for the stereo, and the song "The Hustle" became a big joke among us. She could never remember how to do the dance that went with the song.

My second week back, I folded weight lifting back into the mix. I worked out at the YMCA, on the machines. My muscles responded well and my strength quickly returned. My third week, I rejoined my hockey team, the Pirates. My balance was still very screwed up, but somehow, I was able to play.

***

Soon after I started playing hockey again, I decided to find a really good sub shop in Chapel Hill. I had seen students walk down the street with long subs wrapped in paper, and was determined to find out where they bought them. Finding that sub shop became my quest. Subway franchises abounded, but they did not cut it. I tried independent shops, but they did not sell subs in the long shapes that I had spied the students carrying. Finally, I found Jersey Mike's. As the slogan for Smucker's says, with a name like Jersey Mike's, it had to be good.

Jersey Mike's was located right in the heart of downtown Chapel Hill on Columbia near Franklin Street. The shop had a clean air about it, green Formica tables and televisions suspended near the ceiling. The meats behind the counter looked very good, and the smell of fresh baked bread filled the air.

I decided to try the Italian cold cut sub, number four on the menu. The young man behind the counter began preparing a regular sized sub, but I asked him to make it Giant-sized. I surveyed the accouterments and decided to have lettuce, onion, tomato, banana peppers, oil and vinegar, and spices all lovingly dumped on top. The sub tasted even better than it looked, and I integrated it into my pregame ritual. Every night that I played hockey, I ate a Jersey Mike sub. Soon, the guys there knew exactly what I would order and what toppings I wanted. Dad would later tease me that some people are known at "21" while others are known at Jersey Mike's.

***

Karen came back to visit. When I picked her up at the Raleigh/ Durham airport, it was sunny and eighty degrees. I wore a t-shirt and shorts, sneakers without socks. She thought I looked like a South American playboy. This was a far cry from the last time she saw me.

When I began to play hockey again, I also resumed dating. I began with the young woman that Sherry set me up with, Cathy. On our first date, we met at a coffee shop on Franklin Street. She entered wearing ripped jeans and a grunge t-shirt, her sienna hair swept back in a bun. Despite the generation-x facade, she could just as easily have been wearing a black cocktail dress and pearls. Normally, I don't bring Karen on dates, but she was in town and Cathy didn't mind. The two of them hit it off right from the start. Actually, I was a little depressed that Karen had more in common with her than I did. For example, they had both participated in the same marine biology program on Sanibel Island in Florida. Overall, I was glad that Karen liked her.

On our second date, we went hiking, just the two of us. There was a wonderful state park about ten minutes from my apartment. Jordan Lake stretched for miles and miles. It had a bald eagle nesting area, cormorants, and countless wildlife. Bogart loved going there, and one sunny Saturday, Cathy and I took him.

We had a good time together. It was fascinating to see nature through her eyes. She had studied the environment and pointed out lots of things that I never would have noticed: tadpoles in small puddles of algae, sunken trees that indicated the lake was man-made, turtles. We didn't have a passionate spark, but we enjoyed hanging out.

Life started returning to normal. I went out with Amy Kingman a few more times. I continued to send out the latest version of **Target Market** to any agent that expressed the remotest interest. I hung out with Annette and Jay. They lived in an old Raleigh neighborhood in a house that had a porch with a swing. They liked to just relax out there. On one memorable evening, Jay grilled some Kielbasa that I'm still talking about. I went to a number of very good independent movies. After *Swingers*, I saw *Chasing Amy*, *Ridicule*, and *Kolya*. They were all wonderful. *Chasing Amy* made an especially deep impression. It was about a young comic book artist who falls in love with a lesbian and tries to convert her to heterosexuality. After recommending it to Aaron down in Texas, he told me that it was the story of his friends' lives.

I resumed going to support group. We had speakers that included Ellen Crabtree Brooks, from the Carolina Organ Procurement Agency. Ellen had Scandinavian features and reminded me of an old family friend, Astrid Merget. They had the same color hair, a wheatish blonde. They were both thin, knowledgeable, and easy to talk with.

Ellen described her job. COPA retrieved and allocated organs for transplant. She explained the process that they went through: being alerted that someone was brain dead; notifying the family; explaining the option of organ donation; and getting those organs to people who needed them. She explained brain death to us in a way that I had never heard before. She was incredibly frank. "Brain death is death," she said. When you are brain dead, you are completely done with your organs. Sometimes families see their brain dead relative connected to life support and think that they are still alive and breathing. That is not the case. The machines are merely pumping fluid through a dead body to preserve the organs. The person they knew and loved is no longer there.

We also had a visit at support group from Emily Brimseth, the transplant team's nutritionist. Emily had rounded cheeks and dark hair that fell in bangs. She explained the changes in our diet after transplant. Because of the steroids that we would take, we would need to be on a low sodium diet. This would be an abrupt change for people with CF, who were used to the opposite. She explained that for three months after our operation, we would be on a low-white count diet. This meant that we could eat no fresh fruit or vegetables and no black pepper. All of that contained a fungus called Aspergillus which could be dangerous for immuno-compromised people. Emily explained the fundamentals of good nutrition and taught us how to read the labels on food.

Another speaker was Kelly Jennings. Kelly had received a living donor transplant the prior October. She wore a mask to avoid picking up an infection so it was difficult to see a good portion of her face. Even so, we could tell that she was young. Each of her parents had donated one lobe of their lungs to her. Her voice was still weak because she had been on a ventilator for a very long time, so her parents did most of the talking. But her spirit was loud and very inspiring. She was engaged and planned to get married in the next few months. She was about to move home to Ohio. It was great to see another transplant success story.

Because of support group, by the time of my transplant I knew what to expect on just about every front: pain control; nursing; rehab; nutrition; and medicines. My body chemistry would be very different, and I was ready.

***

My life in Carolina really picked up in mid-March. One night, we organized a group outing from all of the people in the transplant program. Brett, Melissa, Brian, Charity, assorted family members and I went out together. We invited the physical therapists who worked with us and a number of them came. We went to a Mexican dive on Franklin Street. The food was good, but I felt it kicking for an entire weekend. After dinner, we went out and saw Howard Stern's new movie, *Private Parts*. Having grown up in Washington, I remembered listening to him when he was very early on in his career, and parts of the movie brought back memories. I was in junior high back then, and absolutely loved his show. The movie left out some of his best material, like "Jewish Lesbian Karate Expert from New Jersey Dial-a-Date." It was still a great flick. People dismiss entertainers sometimes as not making a meaningful contribution to society, but I have to disagree. During the movie, I looked at the faces of our group, laughing away, and knew what an important service that movie provided: a much needed escape.

Physically, I had now fully recovered. My weight was back to one hundred and fifty-five pounds. My endurance was strong. I could now climb eighty-five flights on a Stairmaster in thirty minutes with no oxygen. And I felt good.

My hockey playing really started to improve. I scored my first assist for the Pirates and my teammates wanted me to score very badly. They encouraged me to hang around the goal so that they could pass me the puck.

On March thirty-first, Annie Downs came to watch me play. As we drove on I-40 together from Chapel Hill to the IcePlex in Raleigh, she shared some big news with me: Michael Ackerman received new lungs that very day and was doing terrific. I got so happy for him that I scored the first goal of my life that night. I was scrapping away in front of the opponents' goal, jostling for position against their defenseman. Our center was very close to me, also in a scrum with the other defenseman. Elias, our left winger shot the puck over, centering it right in front of the net. I redirected it with all of my might and the puck flew past the goalie at his waist level. What a huge thrill. Everyone knew that it was my first goal, and the referee skated over to give me the puck. Later that night, I had an assist.

The following weekend, Amy and Chuck came down to visit. They arrived in time for lunch, so we went to a sub shop on Franklin Street, got take-out, and picnicked on UNC's quad, just across the street. Spring was in full bloom and the sun was out. Friday night, we rolled out the pizza stone they had given me. By now, I sort of knew what I was doing. For example, I no longer rolled out the dough to a width greater than that of the pizza paddle. I did, however, continue to make a complete mess with the cornmeal. Saturday, we went hiking at Jordan Lake and we toured an exhibit of art by Salvador Dali. Saturday night, we had a fajita party. A bunch of friends came over and we pigged out.

On Monday night, April seventh, our hockey team progressed to the semi-finals of our league playoffs. I had an assist in our win. We would be in the Championship game a week later.

Thursday night, I went to a pool party that Summit Hill hosted at the clubhouse. They barbecued hamburgers and hot dogs. Lots of people went and I had a great time. Summit Hill parties had a great reputation for going all out, so attendance was generally very good. At the Christmas party, they served smoked salmon and shrimp.

Friday night, I went dancing with Annette and Jay. They were into Contra dancing, North Carolina's version of square dancing. The dance was in an old building with exposed rafters and a warped wooden floor. It was in the middle of the woods. Once again, I had lots of fun.

Saturday, Cathy had a "bring your own meat" barbecue. Most of the people there were enrolled in Duke Medical School. They were all really nice and it was a very casual evening. Because I wore my beeper, they at first assumed that I was an intern or resident. Many were quite surprised to learn the real reason I wore it. I stayed at Cathy's until after midnight. When it was time to go home, she walked me out to my car and said we should get together soon. She was a huge college basketball fan so I had a surprise for her. I bought a basketball so that we could shoot hoops together. She liked the idea.

Sunday night, I was supposed to go to a CF Foundation fundraiser, an "Evening with The Master Chefs." It would be a seven course feast. I had invited Amy Kingman to go with me. I never made it to the dinner.

CHAPTER 11

❀

The Call

At 6:18, Sunday morning, my phone rang. I woke up and immediately knew what it was. Judy was on the phone. They had a pair of lungs for me, and I should come right over to the emergency room. "Do I have time to walk Bogart?" I asked. That was my only concern. "Hurry," she replied.

I got dressed quickly and out of habit, put my beeper on. I called Dad in Maryland and told him I just got the call. They should come right down. We had a brief conversation. He had the phone numbers for the transplant team and knew where to go in the hospital. I asked him to take care of Bogart as soon as he got to Chapel Hill. Dad assured me that he would take good care of the dog and we hung up.

I took Bogart out on our normal morning walk along the stretch of grass that paralleled the parking lot. While we were out, my beeper went off. The strange thing about it was that it was a musical tone, not straight beeping. The tune it played was "Happy Birthday." That was very odd.

I rushed back inside with the dog and called the number on the beeper. Judy asked me if my Epstein-Barr virus had converted. I told her that I didn't know. She sounded extremely stressed.

I kissed Bogart goodbye, and drove myself to the hospital. On the way, I called Karen up in Boston. She is a very sound sleeper and waking her is not a pleasant task. Dad had tried calling her a few minutes earlier. She had heard the phone ring, but couldn't rouse herself to answer it. When I called, she realized something might be up, so she answered. I told her the scoop, and she said she would head straight to Logan Airport.

I arrived at the emergency room and immediately recognized the triage nurse. She had taken care of me when I arrived with my kidney failure. She had another nurse come and resume her duties at triage so that she could help prep me.

First, she took my vital signs, blood pressure, weight, temperature, and pulse-ox. They were all very good. My pulse-ox was actually 97%. She started an IV in my arm and took some blood. Then she had me begin drinking a gallon of GoLYTELY. This would get me to evacuate my digestive system very quickly. It struck me as ironic that like the story *Alice in Wonderland*, transplant begins with "Drink Me."

A surgical resident gave me a very thorough physical exam, they took x-rays, and the GoLYTELY started to kick in. I had not seen any members of the transplant team, but knew that they were busy getting ready.

After an hour and a half, a nurse from Four Anderson came down to escort me up to the floor. She had a wheelchair but I wanted to walk. No problem.

The nurse and I had a good conversation as we wound our way through the hospital corridors. We got to Anderson Four, the unit where transplant patients go when they leave the ICU. I hadn't finished the entire jug of GoLYTELY, so I carried it with me. As we made our way past the nurses' station, I looked in a room and saw Michael Ackerman. The nurse told me that he would be going home that day. I waved my jug at him and he immediately knew what I was there for. He brightened up and we spoke for a few minutes. I thought he looked great. Like Tom Faraday, he was a new person. No more oxygen. No more exhaustion. It was eight in the morning and he was bright and perky, arguing with a nurse.

We went ten feet further and I recognized a nurse named Michelle. She had been at the Summit Hill pool party Thursday night. It turned out that we were neighbors. She and Annette shared a similar face: beautiful blue eyes and well defined cheeks.

Finally I made it to my room, chugged the rest of the GoLYTELY, and let it do its thing.

Surprisingly, I was relatively calm. Will Crowder, the social worker, says that ninety percent of recipients are calm when they get the call. Part of the reason I remained so calm was that I did not know if my operation was a definite go. Most people get false alarms. They get beeped and at some stage in the process, the transplant is called off. That happens when the donor lungs are not in good condition. They can have an infection or a trauma from the fatal injury. Michael Ackerman had gone through two false alarms that took him all the way to Anderson Four. Some people had made it all the way onto the surgery table before it was called off. As I went through the process, I reserved a little skepticism. Part of me was excited. I kept thinking that "by noon tomorrow, I would have new lungs." The reason I picked noon was that Ian's surgery had ended at noon.

After a while, my nurse left my room. I stared out the window to the rolling hills that extended away from the hospital. Then Judy arrived, decked out in green surgical scrubs and clogs. It was her weekend off, but she had insisted that when my time came, she wanted to be called in. Dr. Egan had objected. He knew how easy it was for people to get burned out and he did not want that to happen to her. But she had told me back in September that she wanted to be there when I got my lungs.

Judy's brow was furrowed. She looked nervous and tried to cover it by concentrating on her clipboard, but I could tell. She told me later that I looked nervous at this point, but I really wasn't.

While Judy was in, a surgeon stopped by my room. Dr. Jones wore a faded, brown leather bomber jacket on top of his green scrubs. He had just come in and his portfolio still hung by its strap over his shoulder. He looked fairly young, tall, and with gold-rimmed spectacles, studious. He told me that Dr. Detterbeck would be doing my transplant, and that he was now in the process of retrieving the new lungs. Dr. Detterbeck was not in the hospital. He was two hours away by plane. Dr. Jones and Judy would be in touch with him to monitor his progress. Dr. Jones told me that Dr. Detterbeck had done a double lung transplant Friday night on a young woman named Nanette Garner.

Michael Ackerman had kicked off a real spurt of transplants. The team had not done any since Mike Hatcher's back in December. That was the nature of their business. It went in cycles of feast or famine.

Dr. Jones explained that he would open me up while Dr. Detterbeck was on his way back to UNC. Opening me up would take about two hours, so they would save precious time once Dr. Detterbeck returned. I had never met Dr. Jones, but again, if the transplant team trusted him, that was fine with me.

At about eleven, a tech from surgery came to pick me up. He asked me to get naked, except for a gown. He had me climb up on a gurney, then put a heated blanket on me. I wanted to walk down to surgery because my legs still worked and I thought it would be bold. He said that at this point it was not allowable. I would have to ride. He was of very good cheer and chatted with me the whole way down. As we went, I realized that his job was not only to get me from one end of the hospital to the other, but also to keep me calm.

We got to pre-op and I met the anesthesiologists. There were three of them. One put a normal IV in my arm. Another started an arterial line in my wrist. This would allow them to monitor my blood pressure and gases very easily. He had a rough time threading the catheter in my wrist, but again, I stayed calm. As he worked, he flirted a little with Judy. That was very amusing.

I made one request to the anesthesiologists: "Please don't let me wake up during the operation." They smiled and promised.

Soon, I was totally prepped. Now we just had to wait for word from Dr. Detterbeck. For the most part, I focused very hard on new lungs. Judy sat in a chair a few feet away from me. She continued to study her clipboard. I tried to chat her up, but she wasn't in a talky mood. So I chatted with the techs who were all very outgoing. I admit that I also scoped out a few of the pre-op nurses.

I knew that I could ask the doctors to give me something to help me relax as I had done in vascular radiology, but I decided that I really didn't need anything.

At about twelve thirty, I received a phone call in Pre-Op. The nurses wheeled the gurney over to the phone and handed it to me. Karen was calling from Washington D.C. She was at Dulles airport where her plane made a brief layover on the way down. The flight attendants let her deplane long enough to call me. I'm amazed that she tracked me down in the hospital. She kept saying that everything would go really well and that she loved me. I kept asking her to make sure the dog was walked. Judy still gives me a hard time about that.

At no time after I got the call did I stop and contemplate the fact that I could die during surgery. Any surgery runs that risk, not just transplant. Deep down, I knew that would not happen to me.

Soon after I hung up the phone with Karen, the techs wheeled me into the operating room. I had never been inside one before. They wheeled my gurney up to the table. It wasn't broad and flat, as I would have expected. Instead, it was narrow and concave, like the bottom half of a steel cocoon. It had narrow boards extending outward for my arms. The tech asked me to take my gown off and slide onto the table. Then he put a new, heated blanket on me. I lay on the table, facing up, still not entirely convinced that the transplant would happen.

I looked around the room, at the monitors, lights, and implements still in their sterile plastic wrappers. Dr. Jones was nowhere to be seen. The anesthesiologists put a mask on my face, and I knew I would soon be asleep. I concentrated really hard on ice-hockey because that's what I wanted to dream about. I often dreamed about hockey games, especially right after playing. I had heard that if you thought about something nice while anesthesia was administered, you would dream about it. Soon I drifted off into a deep sleep. I do not remember dreaming about anything.

Photos

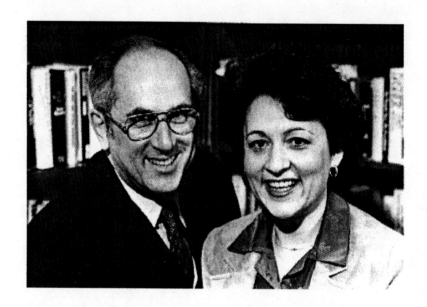

Mom and Dad

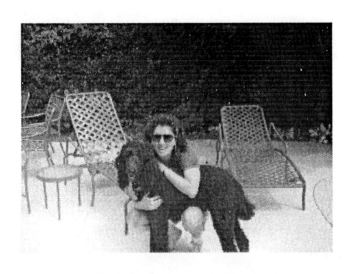

My sister, Karen, and my dog, Bogart

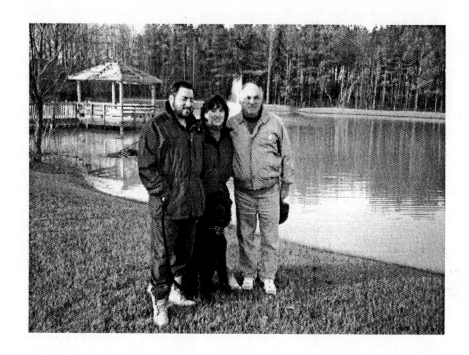

Life in North Carolina before transplant. Charlie, Karen and Dad, with Bogart.

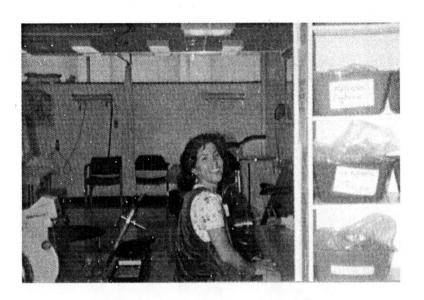

Transplant team physical therapist Annie Downs.

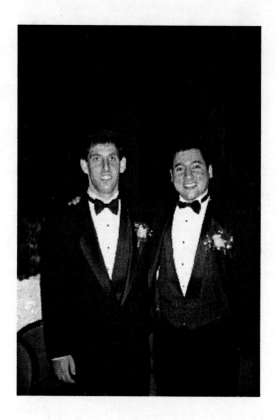

Friend Jon Hefter

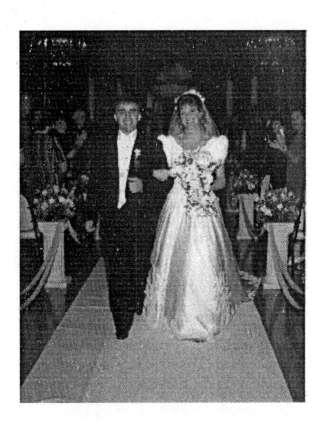

Friends Amy and Chuck Kines

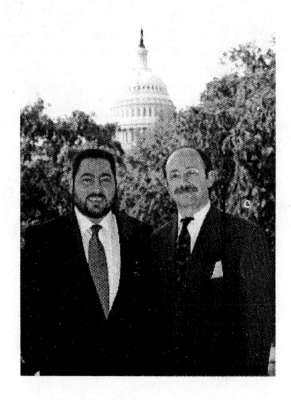

Cousin Jonathan, from Chicago

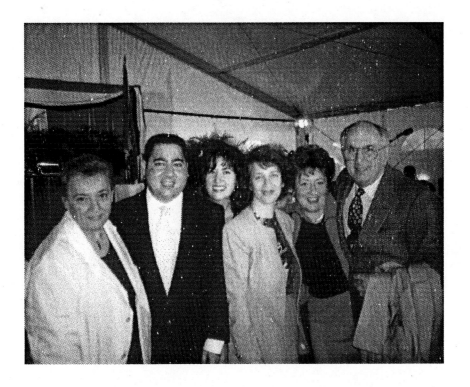

Left to right: Dr. Milica Chernick, Charlie, Karen, friend Dr. Lynn Gerber, Susan and Martin at the National Institutes of Health in Bethesda, Maryland.

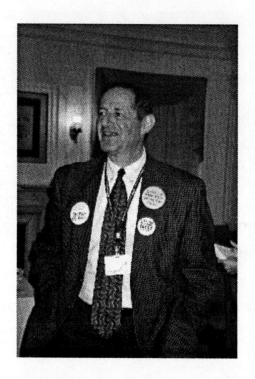

Dr. Beryl Rosenstein of Johns Hopkins Hospital,
shown here promoting flu shots.

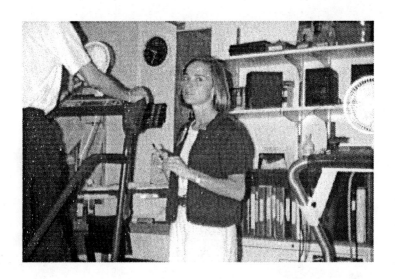

Transplant nurse coordinator and Ironman triathlete Judy McSweeney

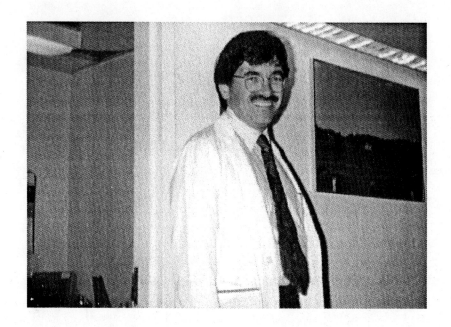

Dr. Tom Egan, lung transplant surgeon.

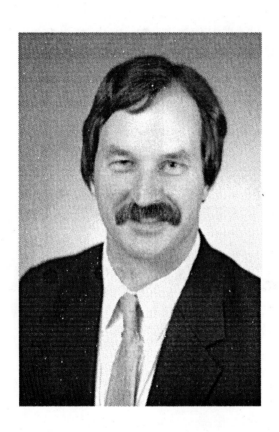

Dr. Frank Detterbeck, my surgeon

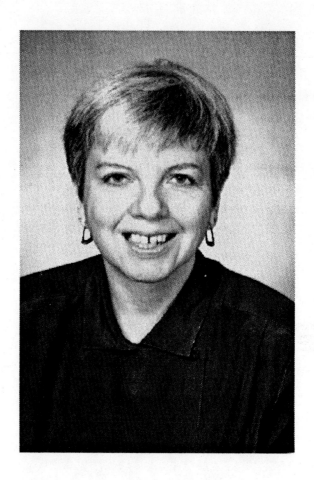

Dr. Linda Paradowski, transplant physician

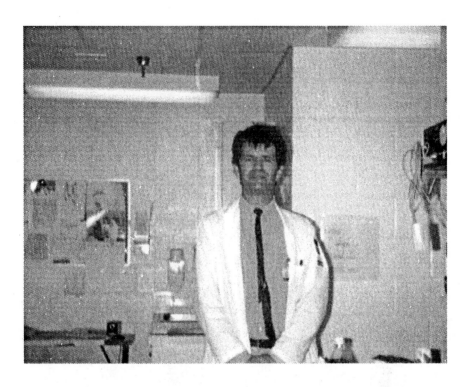

Will Crowder, transplant team social worker

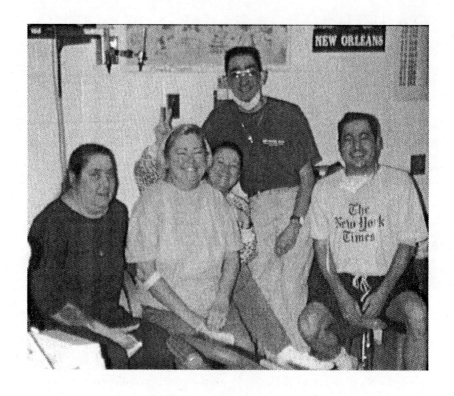

The fighting fivesome, after transplant.
Left to right: Lil "Flash" Shumaker, Mary Ellen "Wild Woman" Smith, Nanette "Lil Bit"
Garner, Michael "Superman" Ackerman, and Charlie "Roadrunner" Tolchin.

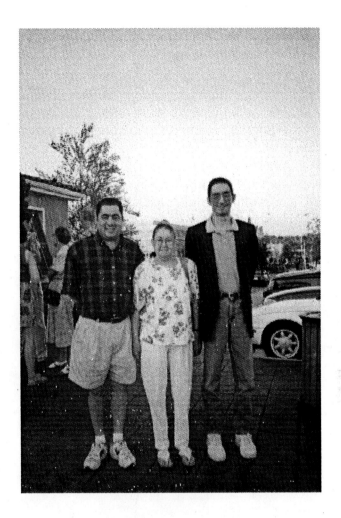

Outside the Macaroni Grill
with Nanette Garner and Michael Ackerman, post transplant.

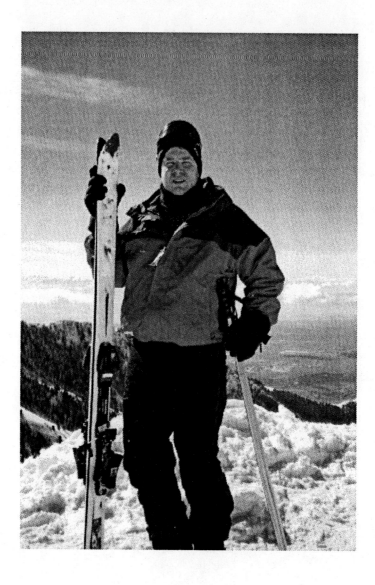

Ian Ferguson enjoying life with new lungs at the top of Snowbasin ski resort in Utah.

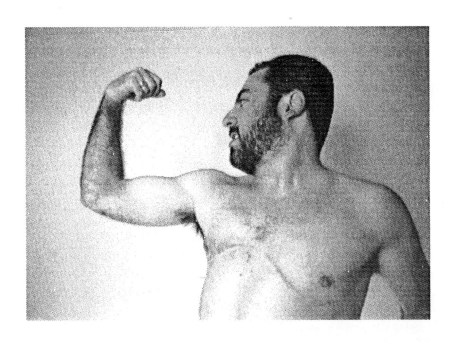

My scar

Chapter 12

Waking up

Mom and Dad arrived at the hospital just after I went into surgery at 12:30 p.m. Karen arrived at three in the afternoon. For the entire day and night, they waited in the ICU waiting room. Every two hours, Judy would call them with an update from the OR. She predicted it would be over by eight p.m.

There were no volunteers in the ICU waiting room so Mom, Dad and Karen took over manning the phone. Like in South Hill, Mom had difficulty understanding the Carolina accents, but she winged it.

Eight rolled around and I was still in surgery. At ten o'clock, they thought it was almost over. Then I started having problems. The surgeons aren't positive what happened, but they have a theory. My donor had been in a terrible accident and suffered numerous broken bones. When that happens, fat can embolize into the donor's bloodstream and travel to the lungs. They think fat had embolized in my donor lungs, and that caused the problem. In addition to that problem, my new lungs were "very wet." When the lungs are transported from donor to recipient, they lie in a saline solution. That fluid seeps into the lungs.

By 12:30 a.m., Dr. Detterbeck, Dr. Jones and Dr. Crowther emerged from the OR. They told my family that the surgery was complete. I was taken to the ICU and at one in the morning, my family got to see me. Karen describes it as the "the most upsetting sight" she had ever seen. I "looked like Frankenstein." During surgery, doctors had put Vaseline on my eyes to keep them from drying out. My family saw only the whites of my rolled back eyes. My skin was yellow, waxy and freezing cold. A bare sheet partially covered me.

My family went into extreme distress. I cannot imagine what it must have been like for them to go through. They clung together in three-way hugs and cried a lot. The family wanted to sleep in a spare room at the hospital but could not find one. The transplant team told them to go home and get some sleep. They came back at 7:30 the next morning. My blood pressure was still terrible but my body had warmed up. The ICU called in one of their best nurses, Ann, to take care of me.

Dad told me that golfer Tiger Woods won the Masters the day before. Even though I was unconscious, I gave the thumbs-up sign. It was the first response I gave to anything and boosted everyone's hopes.

Doctors were unable to wean me off the ventilator. I was still dependent on one hundred percent life support. Doctors feared that so much oxygen would be toxic to me. All day, Dr. Stang sat by my bed, adjusting the ventilator. Dr. Detterbeck could not tell my family whether or not I would survive. Everyone was very upset. Some people privately told my family that I could be on the vent for up to eight weeks. In fact, the prior October, a number of transplant recipients were on vents for six weeks. After that, they recovered and did well.

Up to this point, the doctors kept me sedated. By staying asleep, I could concentrate on healing. While I slept, my family came into my room every hour and spoke to me. They told me that I had a transplant. They told me what day it was, and that I was in the ICU. They assured me that I was safe and that they loved me. Eileen Burker instructed them to tell me all of this to prevent ICU psychosis. She told them to stay positive when they were with me.

Every hour after they left my room, they burst out in tears. At that point, the team really proved the depth of their excellence. Eileen Burker, the team psychologist, and Will Crowder, the social worker, took the family to a private room and offered intensive counseling to them. Judy spent a great deal of time alone with Karen.

My first 24 hours after surgery were extremely rough. I came very close to dying. During this time, only one person believed that I would live: Dr. Paradowski. Nobody else was sure. That included Dr. Detterbeck and Judy.

Dr. Paradowski offered my family the only hope. "We've seen this before, and we know Charlie. He's rocky, but not iffy." "Rocky, not iffy" became the mantra that they clung to. Dr. Paradowski said that she could see me fighting and that my strong physical condition served me well. By late afternoon, my blood pressure started to improve. By Monday night, I started to bounce back and the team started to relax.

On Tuesday, they say I was awake. I have no memory of it. At that point, all of the doctors relaxed. They knew I would make it. My family, though, was still terrified.

Apparently, I was a very happy drunk. I was smiling and in a good mood. Karen would hold my hand and rub my nose. When she would turn to walk away, I would hold onto her tighter. I would smile from behind the vent and laugh when Mom repeated her line: "We're not much, but we're here." She also repeated the phrase: "Don't worry. I'm supervising." Karen says that I was "psychadeliched out."

They had given me a chalkboard to write questions on and I kept repeating the same ones over and over. My short term memory was non-existent.

Soon after I awoke, it became apparent that other people were running my entire body. Nurses would come over and adjust the oxygen flow I inhaled. Actually, they kept lowering it. Nurses decided when I got bathed and when I received doses of medicine. I had absolutely no idea, and didn't care. I had complete trust in them.

In my mind, I woke up from surgery on Wednesday. I knew I was in the ICU. Medical people surrounded my bed and each of their faces bore severe anxiety. I wondered why they looked so nervous. At the foot of my bed, I recognized Dr. Detterbeck. Although I had only met him once before, I knew exactly who he was. I wanted to thank him but I had a ventilator in my mouth which prevented me from speaking. Restraints prevented my hands from ripping out any tubes by accident, so with the fingers of my right hand I motioned him over. Then I reached out to shake his hand.

In the movie *The Terminator*, Arnold Schwarzennegger is sent from the future to present-day Los Angeles. He arrives in a flash of light, in a parking lot, completely naked, kneeling and ready to fight. That is exactly how I felt when I awoke. All of the resources I would need in the world were contained within me.

Things were as I expected they would be for the most part when I awoke. Some people experience ICU psychosis. They are terrified and paranoid. That did not happen to me. I had four chest tubes, a naso-gastric tub, a ventilator, a central-line IV in my neck, EKG monitors, oxygen, a pulse-ox taped to my finger, a urinary catheter, and an arterial line.

A number of things did surprise me. I had never believed Tom Faraday when he described a lack of pain. But when I woke up, I was incredibly stoned on morphine. The doctors had been unable to give me an epidural because of complications during surgery. That would have completely blocked all feeling throughout my torso. The morphine, however, worked just as well. I looked at the wide swath of surgical dressings around my chest tubes and was amazed that things did not hurt. I was amazed that I couldn't feel the urinary catheter. Even so, I refused to look down and see what it looked like. That would have been too much. I was amazed that the ventilator didn't bother me too much. Friends had told me that it was a real pain. For me, though, it was like wearing scuba gear. A nurse held up a mirror so that I could see what the scar looked like. It stretched from one armpit to the other, criss-crossed the entire way by surgical staples. The thought of having them removed became a concern.

I was surprised that doctors had conducted an omental wrap. For most people, they stopped doing that part of the operation. In an omental wrap, surgeons take part of the intestine and thread it up to where the new lungs connect to the old trachea. It serves as a rich supply of blood and is conducive to healing. It means that in addition to the horizontal clamshell, the patient also has a four-inch vertical incision just above the belly button. Patients had always complained that it was more painful than the chest incision.

As I began to wake up, it became clear that there had been some problems. My surgery took place on Sunday. Now it was Wednesday. I had planned to set records, to be up and walking in less than twelve hours. That did not happen.

As my level of consciousness rose, my mood darkened. This must have been due to the combination of steroids and morphine, swirling around inside of me. It must also have been due to some degree of pain that my family says was very blatant.

On Thursday, they tried to get me out of bed. Troy and Billy from physical therapy came. I was still on the ventilator, but that would not be a problem. They switched me to a hand held bag, and then helped me ease off the bed. I thought moving would hurt, but it didn't. Once I got off the bed, though, I struggled to walk only five feet. Billy held onto me from one side, Troy from the other, while a respiratory therapist compressed the bag. The respiratory therapist reminded me of Mike Simpson's mom. She had the same straight salt and pepper hair. I took great comfort in that. I started choking on the ventilator and could not breathe. Karen says that I vomited. They took me back to the bed. I was pissed that I couldn't do more.

Dr. Paradowski ordered the removal of my ventilator. The ICU nurse, Dave, told me later that he argued that it was premature and I would have to go back on the vent. Once the vent came out, I felt better and did not need to go back on it. When the vent came out, I could speak again. It had been in my throat for so long that my vocal chords were shot, but at least I could whisper. My mouth was incredibly dry, and I was very thirsty. I wasn't allowed to drink anything though. My naso-gastric tube was still in and my bowels had not moved. They let me suck on special pink sponges that were soaked in water. Karen would dip it in a cup of water and put it in my mouth. The small trickle of water that it produced felt wonderful. Eventually, they let me suck on ice. Finally, my bowels moved. Hooray.

One by one, the tubes and hoses started coming out. Dr. Paradowski and Dr. Rivera came to remove the n-g tube entirely. I shut my eyes and heard Dr. Rivera's reassuring voice. She held my hand and stroked my hair. The naso-gastric tube stung briefly as the stomach acid laced my throat and nose, but then it was out, and that felt terrific.

Dr. Paradowski said that I could have anything I wanted to drink. What did I want? "Caffeine-free diet ginger ale," I replied. I have no clue why I wanted it. I never drank the stuff. But that's what my taste buds craved. Dr. Paradowski laughed. "Come on, Charlie," she said in her Buffalo, NY, accent. "You can have anything. How about some Cherry Italian Ice." Actually, that did sound good. She got me a paper cup of it, and it was one of the best tasting foods I have ever consumed.

After the vent came out, I had to learn how to cough again. That is yet another strange irony of transplant. Like most CF patients, I had become very skilled at coughing before my transplant. But when doctors install new lungs, they are de-nervated. There is no cough reflex. If a person doesn't learn how to clear mucous again, he can have problems.

The respiratory therapists and nurses tried to teach me how to cough. They used the *NYPD Blue* method. Not the part of the TV show that involved Sherry Stringfellow scampering about in the buff. Rather, the part where they try to get a suspect to confess. One by one, the therapists would stand next to my bed and in a voice like Jimmy Smits, would say: "Anderson Four is much nicer than the ICU. All you have to do to get there is cough." Coughing was just difficult. I felt like one of the criminals banished from the planet Krypton in the first Superman movie. Two of the criminals have laser eyesight that can start fires. The third one has the laser eyes, but they are not hot enough to ignite anything. He keeps staring at things, trying but failing. I kept trying to cough and nothing would happen.

I did have plenty of hiccups. Dr. Detterbeck explained that it was common. The nerves that ran up and down my abdomen had been disrupted.

Strangely enough, the pulse-ox monitor that was taped to my thumb felt very uncomfortable. I asked Judy to remove it. She did and put it on another finger, but my thumb still tingled. During the operation, my thumb had undergone some nerve damage. Dr. Egan later told me that it can be caused by the chest retractors or by lying in an unnatural position for twelve hours.

Every day in the ICU, X-ray technicians came to my room with a portable camera. They wheeled it over my bed, slid the film right under me, and zapped away.

The nurses also started giving me insulin. Two of the drugs I took for immune-suppression, Cyclosporin and Prednisone, made my blood sugar rise. They began checking my glucose regularly, and giving me insulin accordingly. The nurse would walk into my room with a syringe and inject me in places in which I had never been injected before: my thighs and my stomach. Insulin worked best when administered into those large muscles. The first time I saw the nurse approach my stomach with a syringe, I was very concerned. I couldn't speak up quickly enough however, and Dave gave me the shot. It didn't hurt any more than if it were in my arm, so I relaxed.

On Wednesday, they transplanted another patient. It was a boy named Christopher. I didn't know him. His was a living-related transplant. Two of his relatives each donated one lobe to him. That can be done when the patient is much smaller in body size than the two donors. It is usually done as a last resort when it looks as if a cadaver donor will not be found in time. My parents and sister had each wanted to donate a lobe of their lungs to me, but that was not feasible. I heard that Christopher was fighting hard and I began rooting for him.

On Thursday, the nurses gave me a PCA, my own button to control how much morphine I received. Because CF is a digestive disease as well as a lung disease, narcotics can cause severe gastro-intestinal distress. I knew that Michael Ackerman had experienced such problems with the pain meds after his transplant. I feared that if I took too much morphine, my stomach would go postal. But the nurse who gave me the PCA told me to press the button frequently so that I received as much medicine as it would dispense. That was fine with me. I pressed it all the time. I just hoped that my stomach would carry the ball for my incisions.

On Thursday, I became more lucid. I was aware of who was in the room with me. I could converse with people. I was still at the point where I didn't care about too much. I became aware that the television in my room was on all of the time. Morphine played tricks with my mind. At one point, I saw an ad for the movie *The Fifth Element*, a science fiction thriller. Then the morphine kicked in and I dozed off. I dreamt that I was in the movie with incredible detail. I woke up a little unnerved. I stared at the wall and saw a few weird shapes in the Tarheel Blue paint. I still remember seeing a skull. It didn't scare me.

As I lay there in the ICU, I thought about Cape Cod. The air up there is wonderful, clear and unpolluted. Wind off the Atlantic carries the scent of scrub pine mixed in with very sweet sand. Every summer when we cross over the bridge onto the peninsula, I roll down the windows to the car and stick my head out like Bogart. What would it be like to inhale the Cape air with new lungs? I was very eager to find out.

Just outside my room, work crews were using jack hammers on a section of the roof. That drove me crazy. My room seemed to shake from the vibrations, and the noise was unbearable.

On Thursday, I began sitting up in a chair for one hour stretches. It was exhausting, but would help get my lungs opened up.

As people came into my room, they all commented on how pink my nailbeds were. With CF and many other lung diseases, the poor supply of oxygen changes the look of the finger tips. It leads to clubbing, in varying amounts. Instead of appearing normal with flat nailbeds, clubbed fingers are rounder, and almost bubble around the nail. The nailbeds also can become blue instead of pink. I could never tell by looking at my own nails whether they were blue or pink. The change in hue would always occur too slowly for me to notice. After my transplant, when everyone commented on how nice and pink my fingernails were, I could not see it.

On Thursday, Mary Ellen, the wild woman, got new lungs. I was so happy when I heard the news.

Friday, when the physical therapists came to take me walking, I could do a lap around the entire ICU. My family was amazed at how Troy and Billy untangled all of the lines that connected me to machines and kept them straight. The therapists loaded the Pleur-Evacs onto a wheelchair and I pushed it just like in the slides that Annie had shown me. Now when I left my room, I had to wear a surgical mask to protect me from all of the germs in the hospital air. I would have to wear it every time I entered the hospital for the entire first year after my transplant. Because my immune system was deliberately reduced, I was now at much greater risk for contracting many infections.

On Friday, my urinary catheter came out. Dave, my nurse, came into my room and told me it was time. I was still pretty stoned, but I worried that if I couldn't pee yet, they would have to put another one back in. It stung briefly as it came out, but luckily, my bladder started pumping on its own. That made me extremely happy.

Friday, I was able to walk two laps around the ICU. They let me start drinking more, and I was finally able to cough. It was weak, but it counted. Now I was alert enough to be bored. The TV carried two channels and my choices were auto racing and "America's Funniest Home Videos." Neither offered enough distraction.

My family took to bringing the nurses large boxes of donuts. It was how they expressed gratitude. When my family was late in visiting me, the nurses would jokingly ask me where the donuts were.

On Saturday, Dr. Paradowski ordered me moved down to Anderson Four. She personally pushed my wheelchair. Again, they called in a special nurse to take care of me, Carrie Prascak. Carrie arrived mid-afternoon. She was about my age and very cute. She grew up in Milwaukee, loved pro football, and had the same laugh as the cartoon character "Huckleberry Hound."

Carrie got me settled into my room on Anderson Four. She announced that I smelled really bad and insisted on bathing me. That was fine with me. The nurses in the ICU had given me sponge baths and the warm water had always felt very good. So Carrie moved me over to the sink and worked her magic.

I still had four chest tubes in. They stretched from my chest to the two Pleur-Evacs, and from the Pleur-Evacs into wall suction devices. That helped keep the pressure in my lungs full. Essentially, I was stuck to the wall with about eight feet to move around.

On Saturday, I ran a low grade temperature. Doctors thought that it might be rejection, which affected most people at UNC within the first week. They blasted me with a super high dose of steroids. The IV form of Prednisone was called Solu-medrol. The first day, I was given one thousand milligrams. For the next two days, I received five hundred. That made my chest break out with terrible acne. It looked like the pimpled surface of a basketball. The acne was very uncomfortable and itched terribly.

That Saturday, Mom, Dad and Karen went to a festival on Franklin Street. It was called "Apple Chill." Mom bought me a stuffed animal, a blue frog. I liked it, but felt a little old to be playing with stuffed animals.

***

The stress from the ordeal made my family start fighting.

Soon after I arrived on Anderson Four, it became apparent that the family was in crisis. Mom and Dad were not getting along with Karen. Karen felt that they were not vigilant enough in washing their hands when they were around me. She pointed this out to them constantly because she thought they were a real danger to my health. They had a rough time adjusting to the new regimen because they had always treated me like a normal person and it had served me very well.

Even a loving and supporting family like ours had its limits. Mom and Dad felt that the touch and go part of the transplant was over, that I was on the mend, and that Karen could now go back to Boston. She would not hear of it. So they asked me what I wanted. I said "Karen stays." That turned out to be a very good thing.

CHAPTER 13

❀

Recovery-Week One

On Anderson Four, my recovery began to accelerate. One by one, the IV pole carried fewer bags of medicine. It went from carrying four pumps to three to two. The doctors lowered the dose of morphine I received with my PCA. They usually did not tell me when they did so, but my level of discomfort remained about the same. They would ask me what my pain was on a scale of one to ten.

I had always expected some pain after transplant. I anticipated it to be somewhere between how I felt after my first day playing ice-hockey and being hit by a Cessna. While it was much worse than how I felt after hockey, for the most part, I was not in a great deal of pain. As the second week wore on, however, my chest tubes started to hurt. They didn't hurt all of the time, just if I moved in certain ways. Each tube extended eighteen inches inside me from just below my rib cage to the upper lobes of my new lungs. The two tubes on my right side hurt the most. If I extended my right arm out, a searing pain would shoot through my torso. When that happened, I reflexively yelled out in pain. So, I began using only my left arm.

The surgical dressings for my chest tubes had to be changed every two days to prevent infection. That was very uncomfortable for me. Doctors had not shaved my chest or stomach before the surgery for fear that a nick could get infected. As a result, layers of cloth surgical tape with its heavy adhesive clung hard to my body. At my request, the nurses and nursing students that changed the dressings began using an adhesive remover called Detachol. It helped some but the procedure still required a significant amount of tugging on very sensitive skin around the chest tubes. The adhesive remover smelled like super-sweet, pumpkin-flavored alcohol. The scent of it turned my stomach.

One day, Troy came to my room. Out of the blue, he raised one of my arms above my head to check my mobility. He gave no warning. If he had, I would have told him not to because of my chest tube soreness. My mobility was fine. The movement hurt my chest tubes a great deal. They ached for about a day after that incident.

On Monday, I underwent my first bronchoscopy. That had been Ian's biggest fear before transplant. I never thought about it. When my time came, I was a little nervous, but barely. I was still under the influence of serious morphine so I did not care about anything too much. A nurse wheeled me to the bronch suite in the tower part of the hospital. My family followed along. Again, they looked nervous.

Judy helped me onto the bronch table. It was heavy and mechanized, with a padded mattress covered by a sheet. The table was bent in half so that I could sit up. Judy injected something into one of my IV ports and said "goodnight Charlie." The next thing I remember, I was told it was over and my lungs looked good. Judy gave me a photo taken during the bronch. It showed the connection sites where my old trachea met my new lungs. The bronch was like an alien abduction, where no time elapsed. If that's what bronchs were like, they would be no problem.

★★★

The Jewish Holiday of Passover fell that Tuesday. It is my favorite holiday, not just because of the outstanding food, but also because the lesson is so relevant to modern life. The holiday celebrates the Jews' exodus from Egypt. It is about being a stranger in a foreign land. That is how we were in North Carolina, strangers in a foreign land. Like the woman in the furniture rental store, North Carolinians are by nature, friendly, outgoing and hospitable, in essence always fulfilling the spirit of Passover.

One of the respiratory therapists, Lynn Shapiro, embodied that spirit. She knew that we were Jewish and suggested to her friend, Sema Lederman, that she help us celebrate. We had never met Sema, but she brought us a plate for a Seder dinner to my hospital room. She then invited Mom, Dad, and Karen to her house for a Passover dinner. They accepted and had a marvelous time.

Later that night, I received a phone call in my room. It was Bill Safire, back in Bethesda. Our family had celebrated Passover at his house every year since we moved to Maryland. Although I could not speak, Dad held the phone to my ear and Bill told me how they had prayed for me and were thinking about me.

***

Back on Anderson, life developed into a routine. Every day I would ask how Christopher, Nanette, and Mary Ellen were doing. I had not met Christopher or Nanette but we all followed each others' progress. Each morning at six, a surgical resident would make the first round of the day. Soon after, all of the doctors would come by together. The door to my room had a glass window and I could always hear them talking outside just before they entered. When I heard their voices, I would think to myself "ask not for whom the bell tolls…"

Early each morning, a phlebotomist would come by to draw my blood. By eight, x-ray would call to have me sent down. With all of my chest tubes and my IV pole, it took a nurse and an assistant to get me down there. Because my chest tubes were still dependent on suction from the wall unit, when I traveled I had to use portable suction pumps. They ran on batteries that would last a total of fifteen to twenty minutes. That's how long we had to get me down to x-ray and back before the pumps would sputter out and die.

They would wheel me into x-ray and then with all of my chest tubes, I would hug the metal sheet that held the film as the machine did its job. I would wait until the tech checked the film to make sure it developed properly, before heading back upstairs. When they stuck the film into the light box, I could see my new lungs. I could see the wire that held my sternum in place. I could see the chest tubes wend their way through my torso. And I could see the staples that snaked across my incision. It all looked very cool.

It was at x-ray one morning that I first met Nanette. Our wheelchairs were pulled alongside each other like Navy ships as we waited in the hallway. She recognized me and said "hey" in a thick Carolina accent. I was still fairly stoned and did not recognize her. When she introduced herself, then I knew. She did not look well. Although she had been discharged from the ICU after two days, she had endured unrelenting difficulties with nausea and anemia. Most mornings, we were able to see each other in that hallway and chat briefly. Her dad was usually with her. He slept in a chair in her room every night.

After x-ray and breakfast, the physical therapists would come by to take me walking. One week after my operation, Annie came to take me to work out on a treadmill. The main physical therapy department did not have a wall suction unit for my Pleur-evacs so therapists converted a small storage room on Anderson Three into a tiny gym. I walked very slowly, one mile an hour. I was sore, and a little amazed at how much strength I had lost in just seven days. When I didn't go to the Anderson Three treadmill, the therapists would have me do laps around Anderson Four. They loaded my Pleur-evacs onto a wheelchair and got the portable suction pumps fired up. I would put on a mask and be off. At first, I could only do one lap, slowly.

The physical therapists would come by in the afternoon for a second session. I was determined to complete at least one more lap than my previous session. If I did four laps in the morning, I tried to do five in the afternoon.

On one occasion, the therapists got caught up with other patients and could not come to see me. I went into a panic and asked Karen to call Annie. Annie made sure that someone came to take me walking. I knew that PT was the only way I was going to get better, to get my new lungs working at one hundred percent, to get my chest tubes yanked, and to get the heck out of the hospital. Later, Annie told me that patients never call asking for more PT.

The respiratory therapists came to work with me on a device called an incentive spirometer. It consisted of a plastic mouthpiece attached to a hose, which led into an air chamber. The chamber held a blue plunger and was marked by volume of CCS. By clasping one's lips around the mouthpiece and inhaling, the plunger rose. The goal was to lift the plunger as high as possible in the air chamber. That helped build up the diaphragm muscles and open up the small airways. My new lungs did not come installed at one hundred percent function. It would take months for them to fully inflate. The respiratory therapists asked me to take ten deep breaths with the spirometer. It was very hard work and I could barely lift the plunger 500 CCS per breath.

I began to eat that first week on Anderson Four. A little at first, then my appetite kicked in. I had to learn a new diet. Now I could not eat any black pepper. I could not eat any fresh fruit or vegetables. I could not eat anything high in sodium. One day, Amy Kingman came to visit during dinner. She was working on another unit and had heard about my transplant. She stopped by to see if I wanted to join her for Chinese carry-out with some of her friends. I was already working my way through a very big spaghetti dinner. I was very hungry and happily stuffing my face. It was good to see her, and she kept me company while I ate.

One night, a nurse came into my room with my first oral dose of Cyclosporin. This lowered my immune system to prevent my body from rejecting my new lungs. Up until this point, doctors had given it to me intravenously. Now that I could eat and drink, they wanted me to ingest it orally. The brand name of Cyclosporin was Neoral. Each pill came in a sealed tin foil packet. When the nurse brought me my Neoral, she opened up the tin foil packets and placed them on my tray. Then she left. An overpowering smell emanated from the pills and filled the entire room. It was so bad that it made me nauseous. It smelled like a combination of burnt tennis shoe rubber and concentrated cod-liver oil. I had to take the pills, but I could not even bring myself to go near them. For an hour, I sat on the edge of my bed, getting more and more upset. The thought of placing those pills in my mouth nearly brought me to tears.

Finally, I grabbed one, placed it under my tongue and gulped down a swig of water. The pill tasted far worse than it smelled. The water tasted foul as did the paper cup. My gut wrenched and I almost vomited. There were four pills in all, and I honestly don't know how I managed to consume them.

After that, I dreaded my next dose of Neoral. After a few days, I learned to take it a little better. A good friend of mine quit smoking by drinking an overpowering grape juice every time he felt the need to light up. I used the same grape juice to mask the smell of the Neoral. My nurse, Fe, would pour me a huge cup of grape juice. I would hold it under my nose and inhale a huge whiff of it so that the smell coated my nostrils. Then I would take a huge gulp of it so that it coated my mouth. Then I held it under my nose again so that it was all I could smell. As I held it there, Fe would quickly open a packet of Neoral, I would pop it in my mouth and swallow more grape juice. Even doing all of that, my gut would still wrench every time I swallowed a pill. It was as if my body considered it a poison and instinctively rejected it.

Some of my friends have told me that they cannot taste Neoral at all. The smell never bothered them. Kim Brown can swallow the pills without any water at all. This blows my mind.

Every few hours, a nurse would come in to check my blood sugar. That seemed to be a rising problem. As I ate more, my diabetes became more pronounced. My sugar was always elevated. They would give me insulin to lower it.

The week that I arrived on Anderson Four, Judy began an intensive education program with me. First, she gave me a transplant notebook. I had received an older version of it when I first met the transplant team back in 1993. Judy asked me to read the book and learn everything in it before I went home. She gave me a three ring binder that contained my new schedule of medicine along with a green, plastic bucket that held bottles of all my new medicines. I would have to commit to memory my new schedule of pills, what they all were, and their unique qualities. She brought in a bag filled with forms for the blood lab and x-ray. Whenever she ordered tests, I would have to fill out my own forms and bring them to the proper department. She brought me a portable PFT machine and an automatic blood pressure cuff so that at home I could check myself every morning.

Her timing turned out to be unfortunate. When people are given Solu-medrol, there is a risk of seizures. To prevent that, they are given a drug called Atavan for eight days. In addition to being an anti-convulsive, it is also a mild sedative. Within a half-hour of taking an Atavan, I would get very drowsy. My eyelids would droop and I would drift off. Judy seemed to time half of her lessons to just after I received Atavan. She would begin to talk and my eyelids would start to droop. Then she would get mad that I wasn't paying attention. Other times, she would come in and start a lesson when I did not have any Atavan. During those instances, she invariably would make a comment like: "I can see you fading fast here." I would be wide awake. We laugh about it now but at the time it was very frustrating.

Carrie, who had moved me down to Anderson with Dr. Paradowski, and I became very close. I looked forward to her shifts. We would talk about lots of things and seemed to be on nearly identical wavelengths. We grooved to the point where it seemed as if we had known each other for a long time. When she was around me, she would giggle in her Huckleberry Hound way constantly and act a little bit nervous. Every time she left my room, my family would immediately tell me that she liked me. This came during the only two week period in modern history when I was not actively dating. I was very focused on getting better.

In addition to Carrie, there were a number of fine nurses who took care of me on Anderson Four.

Fe worked nights. She was very laid back, like the clinic nurse on the TV show "Northern Exposure." Every night, she would bring over my toothbrush and a container to spit in.

Betty was a nursing assistant. She had a degree in communications and was preparing for graduate school in speech pathology. She was out and out stunning but completely unaware of it. I could not look at her without thinking "Betty Grable." Betty would help me wash. I would sit in a chair by the sink and she would take a warm wash cloth and scrub my back. It was one of my only pleasures.

Desiree grew up on the Virginia-Carolina border and spoke in a thick accent. I loved listening to her talk. She wore gold-rimmed spectacles and looked thoughtful. She went running and was clearly in outstanding shape. Like Judy, she had magnificent neck muscles. I enjoyed flirting with her.

Kerri was a fellow hockey psycho. We talked about that often. The playoffs had begun while I was in the ICU. This year, the Washington Capitals did not make it so I couldn't root for them. But I did get to watch lots of hockey on TV. It was on almost every night. Because Dr. Paradowski was a Buffalo Sabres fan, I mostly rooted for them. But because of Mario Lemieux, I also rooted for the Penguins. I always admired the way he fought cancer and came back to play professional hockey again. It was the last season of his career and I watched him play his last professional game against the Philadelphia Flyers.

One night, Lucy took care of me. She was on loan from another unit. She had been the nurse who took care of me during my evaluation twenty-eight months earlier and secretly told me how talented Dr. Stang was. Other nights, Sherrie took care of me. She had great hair and Mom and Karen talked hairdressers with her. Cheryl took care of me on weekend nights. She was into investing and we talked about stocks.

There was one strange quality to all of the nurses. Usually they all share the same hand lotion and soap. On Anderson Four, they all smelled as if they wore the same perfume, "Vanilla Beans." I cannot smell it without thinking of them.

My sleep patterns went haywire on Anderson Four. I could not doze off until well after midnight and I would be up for the day by three-thirty or four at the latest. Will Crowder told me that this was common. As I lay awake in bed, I thought about hockey. What would it be like to play with new lungs? What would it be like to play without getting short of breath? What would it feel like to skate fast and stop opponents from breaking away down the ice, to skate faster than them, to strip the puck away from them? I imagined my legs whipped up into a cartoonish blur.

As I lay awake, I also imagined what it would be like to return to work and reclaim my advertising career. What would it be like to be able to work a full day and not be exhausted at the end, as I had been at Circuit City? What would it be like to spend my days in a real advertising agency, not the fictional one that I created in my writing? What would it be like to get my own apartment once again?

I could not wait.

I did not think about the risk of rejection that I would face as I moved forward in my life, or about the risk of dangerous infections.

When the surgical residents made their rounds at six, I would already be out of bed, sitting up in my chair. Soon they started checking on me earlier. They would do rounds on me at five to get me out of the way. I never asked for medicine to help me sleep for a few reasons. First, I felt that I was taking enough pharmaceuticals to choke a horse. Second, I feared that too much narcotics would give me stomach problems. So far, though, my gut was doing fairly well.

I had only one problem in that regard. For years, my routine CF meds included a drug called Colace. It is a stool softener, or laxative. With CF, the thick mucous in our lungs can make our stool very hard like cement. Colace prevents that from happening. When my bowels awoke after surgery, I reminded the doctors that I needed Colace. They kept forgetting to order it. Things were starting to get painful. I was afraid that my bowels might get blocked up. Every day I asked for it, at least twice. It never came. Finally, I asked Karen to retrieve my own supply from home and she smuggled it in. After that I felt fine and dandy.

Going to the bathroom reflected my utter lack of inhibition. It was a bit of an endeavor with chest tubes so I needed help. It would be painful if I reached down to carry the Pleur-evacs so I needed a nurse to help me move them. The nurse would stretch my tubes from the wall to the Pleur-evacs to the bathroom. I would go in, do my business, and hit the call button when I finished. Just a week earlier, I did not want to get naked before going down to the OR. Now, I did not care one whit who helped me answer the call of nature.

One day when I got into the bathroom, I dropped my sweat pants and boxer shorts, and noticed that my groin was not in the same condition it was when I entered the hospital. Half of my pubic hair was shaved, in a diagonal slant. It looked like Flash Gordon's logo. I had completely expected this, but forgotten about it. The reason for shaving is so that if surgeons need to access a large vein in the groin during the surgery, they can in a moment's notice. Later, I would joke with Judy about it that I was surprised that she did not etch her initials into the stubble. Of course that made her blush as I knew it would.

There were two surgical residents assigned to my case: Dr. Cornwell and Dr. Ball. Dr. Jones supervised them and made rounds, but they attended to the minutiae of my case. They were both in their first year. They both practically lived at the hospital. And they were both very good doctors.

Dr. Cornwell was an exceptional listener and she was gentle but honest. One day, when I asked how Christopher was doing, she told me that he had passed away. I knew that he had a very rough time, and the transplant team worked very hard to get him to pull through. When he died, it tore up the doctors and nurses—I could see it in their faces. His family members who donated their lobes to him were also very depressed. Sometimes I could see them walking on Anderson Four, trying to recover from their own surgeries.

Dr. Ball was more intense than Dr. Cornwell. Every morning, when they made rounds on me, they checked the fluid output from my chest tubes into the Pleur-evacs. As long as they continued to drain, the tubes would have to remain inside me. One day, Dr. Jones thought that maybe the tube entry sites were not sealed properly with Vaseline. It might be causing a leak. Dr. Ball changed the dressings, meticulously laying down each new layer of tape.

Sometimes, the phone in my room would ring. That caused problems. I could not reach it within three or four rings. If I did answer it, my voice was so shot from the ventilator that callers could not decipher my words. Finally, I gave up answering it.

✶✶✶

One morning, my x-rays showed an infiltrate in my lungs. This was fairly common and doctors monitored it closely. When my family arrived to visit me that day, they asked the nurses at the station for an update on my health. One nurse got them very scared by saying that I had pneumonia and was very sick. They rushed into my room and wanted to know what was going on. I said that things were fine, as I thought they were. But my family did not believe me and relayed what the nurse told them. I said: "She's a nurse. Go find a doctor and talk about it with him or her before you get really upset."

They tracked down Dr. Ball. He alleviated their concern immediately. He said it was no big deal. Then Karen flexed that brain power of hers. She had not been fully informed about transplant beforehand. She had been to a few support groups, but did not know a great deal about the nuts and bolts of the operation. As soon as she landed in Chapel Hill, she saturated herself with transplant. She learned an impressive amount, to the point where she fully understood what the doctors where saying. Now she grilled Dr. Ball. "Would his incentive spirometer be helpful in clearing up the infiltrate?" she asked him. "That *is* a good idea," he replied. "Have him do it every fifteen minutes, when the commercials come on."

Later, she made a keen observation. "I think your doctor is your next door neighbor." Dr. Ball had lived next door to me at Summit Hill for five months but I did not recognize him. I lived in apartment K-5. He was in K-4. I had seen him only twice during that time, when he was driving off. He was very surprised to learn that we were neighbors. "You're the one with the dog that stares out the window and barks at everybody?" he asked. "Yup. That's Bogart," I said with pride.

Toward the end of the week, my family noticed that I seemed to be in more pain. They raised the issue with Dr. Cornwell. "Oh, we can't have that," she told them. She then ordered more morphine for me.

***

After being on Anderson Four for a week, cousins Ruthie and Jonathan flew in from Chicago to visit. They entered my room wearing Groucho Marx glasses, the kind with a nose and mustache attached. I was really happy to see them. So was my family. The stress that they had been under really showed and Ruthie and Jonathan offered them a wonderful distraction.

They went out to dinner and saw some of the sights. They visited me every day, but were very sensitive not to stay too long. Dad was terrific about that throughout. I did not care too much who was there or for how long. But Dad made sure I was not over-taxed entertaining people.

Along with Mom, Dad, and Karen, Ruthie and Jonathan joined me when I did laps around Anderson Four. I would push the wheelchair with the Pleur-evacs and one of them would push my IV pole. Now I tried to get walking as much as possible, three and four times a day. Jonathan told me that it was the most focused he has ever seen anybody. Karen says that whoever pushed the pole for me struggled to keep up, especially as I swerved around the turns.

Before they went home to Chicago, Jonathan gave me a videotape that he had made. He wouldn't tell me what was on it, but strongly urged me to have a nurse wheel in a VCR so that I could watch it. I just was not able to concentrate too much, so I held off on finding a VCR.

CHAPTER 14

Recovery-Weeks Two and Three

Immediately after my transplant, Amy Kines jumped into action. She was in charge of my phone list. Before I left Maryland, I gave her a list of about fifty people to call when I received new lungs. It had been such a thrill for me to get a call the day of her wedding telling me that Ian had just left the OR and was doing great. I wanted my friends to share in that wonderful news as soon as possible. I expected to do just as well as Ian, but that was not the case immediately following my operation. It was not the case when Amy contacted everyone. My friends each received a scary call accurately describing my situation. Poor Amy ended up living on the telephone in the ensuing days, calling them repeatedly as I began to recover.

As soon as they got the call from her, my friends and family offered an overwhelming amount of support. I received hundreds of get well cards, all of which I kept. As I received them, Dad taped them up. Soon they covered a wall. My friend Eve made a wonderful card that transposed my face onto a hockey player's body. Looking at that reminder of who I was motivated me a great deal. The young woman that succeeded Karen as editor of the Howl, Julie Fanburg, created a wonderful humor book for me. She glued in a toy doctor's kit, a pack of spinach, and dirty jokes. She also inserted the latest *Playboy* tribute to the women of the Atlantic Coast Conference. It was hysterical. Aaron and Leslie Roffwarg sent me a pile of magazines and a book of truly tasteless cartoons. One day Mom picked it up and started to flip through it. I told her that she would probably be very offended by the content and she might not want to continue reading, but she insisted. She ended up laughing through every page. Cathy, whose party I attended the night before the transplant, was a very talented artist. She made a painting for me of a colorful, abstract yin and yang.

My friends wanted to come down to visit me, but we really discouraged that. I just wanted to focus on healing. They did start praying for me like crazy. Mrs. Fisher, my old soccer coach led a prayer circle.

Sherry, who cleaned my house and was a minister, went into prayer overdrive. She had people praying for me all over the state. She took care of Bogart for me while I was in the hospital. That way, my family did not have to worry about him.

Many doctors came by to see me, even ones that did not take care of me. One night, Dr. Knowles came by with a young med student. We talked for a while and then they left. He later told me that the student was his own son.

Dr. Yankaskis came by and talked with Karen and me for an hour. I was fairly stoned, but I remember it clearly. He was fascinating. He described his work before he went to medical school. In a prior incantation, he was an aeronautical engineer. As a hobby, he still piloted his own plane. He had designed the cockpit of the Blackhawk helicopter. He described how he applied his engineering background to medicine. He said that some professors teach sheer memorization, but he teaches problem solving.

Dr. Yankaskis told me about the CF Fundraiser that I missed the night of my transplant. He said that he stood before the crowd and told everyone that I would not be able to make it that night because I was getting new lungs. He then presented me with a program from the event that everyone signed.

He had actually been in the OR and retrieved my old lungs for research purposes. He said that they looked pretty bad and that he had no idea how I crossed the street, much less played ice-hockey. He did note that there was one small area of healthy pink tissue in the upper right lobe which surprised him.

Dr. Yankaskis also told me about his wife. Bonnie Yankaskis was a physician and researcher at UNC as well. She focused on breast cancer. He swelled with pride as he described her. I hoped that someday when I got married, I admired my wife as much as he did.

At the end of our conversation, I vomited. I had received an IV medicine called CytoGam that day, a drug that prevented CMV, or Cytomegalo Virus.

I had never placed much value in get well cards. After all, they were a reminder that I was not healthy. That was the last thing I always wanted to hear. My family always dissuaded people from sending me things in the hospital. For the few that were adamant, they said: "send him a pizza." But now, the cards were welcomed. I was really glad to know that all of these people were looking out for me in the hospital, and that all of my friends back home were pulling for me there.

Congressman Gary Ackerman of New York surprised our family. We had gotten to know him over the past few years. While I was in the ICU, where there are no phones in the patient rooms, he tracked Dad down to offer his support. We still do not know how he found us.

***

My chest tubes continued to be a problem. By the end of that second week, they hurt much more. Now they hurt when I moved, if I stood up or sat down. They hurt when I got into or out of bed. At this point, I avoided my bed altogether. The mattress sagged and was very uncomfortable. My room had a La-Z-Boy type recliner and I spent most of my time sitting on it. Instead of going to bed at night, I would sleep in that chair.

Every morning when Dr. Cornwell and Dr. Ball checked the Pleur-evac output from the previous day, I hoped that they would announce good news. It did not come. Liquid still drained. My other friends had been out of the hospital within two weeks. Here I was, not going anywhere. I began to feel like Bill Murray in the movie *Groundhog Day*. Each day I woke up to the disturbing reality that it was identical to yesterday. I began to suspect that my chest tubes were never going to come out.

Each year, the transplant program had a big picnic. It served as a homecoming for all of the graduates of the program, and a motivator for people waiting. It was held in a park in the next town over, Carrboro. Will would barbecue hamburgers and hot dogs, and everyone brought a dish. This year's picnic was scheduled for May first. I wanted to attend it very badly. I wanted to be out of the hospital in time for the picnic.

At the ten day mark, a med student came to take out my staples. Her name was Siobman and she had been making rounds with the surgeons. I was nervous, but she explained that unlike paper staples that curled back on themselves, surgical staples went directly in and out. They stayed straight. She had a small pliers-type device and began removing them. It did not hurt at all. The skin along my incision was still very numb, so that may have helped. After the staples were all removed, she placed steri-strips across the incision. These were two-inch bits of very strong tape. It was like strapping tape used for shipping, the kind with twine embedded in the plastic.

***

My diabetes continued to be a problem. The transplant team disagreed with the surgical team as to how to treat it. With insulin, there are a number of options. There is NPH, or long acting insulin that works for twelve hours; 70/30, a mixture of long acting and short acting insulin; R, which acts in the medium range of about five hours; and Humalog, which is referred to as "rocket fuel" because it kicks in within ten minutes and burns up in about three hours. I knew none of this at the time of my transplant.

Insulin can be used in a number of ways. It can be used to lower blood sugar that is already elevated, or it can be used to prevent blood sugar from rising. This turned out to be the crux of the disagreement. The surgical team wanted to use insulin to lower my glucose, while the transplant team wanted to use it to prevent my glucose from rising. At one point, Judy and Dr. Ball got into an argument about it right in front of me. Dr. Ball turned to me and said: "While you're here, you're our responsibility." To which Judy countered: "After you leave here, we will be taking care of you forever."

They were all smart people and I felt clueless. I got mad because their disagreement meant that a nurse came into my room every two hours to prick my finger and give me a shot. None of the nurses checked my glucose the way Judy taught me to. Judy showed me how to prick my fingers on the side, where there are less nerve endings than on the pads. Every nurse grabbed my finger and pricked smack dab in the middle of the pad. My fingers were starting to hurt and my skin began to bruise. It seemed excessive and I complained. They cut back the glucose tests to every four hours but still did not resolve their fundamental difference.

Week Three

Ruthie and Jonathan flew back to Chicago Sunday afternoon. Dad went back to Maryland on Monday morning. I was on the mend and he could go back to work. His company had been very supportive. The boss of *The Hill*'s parent company made sure he knew that he could stay in North Carolina as long as was needed. From that point on, he would fly back and forth, visiting us every weekend.

By now, I had my medicine schedule memorized. When it was time for a dose, I opened a bottle and took a pill. Once they knew that I had it memorized, the nurses disinvolved themselves. The day started with my prednisone and Cyclosporin at eight a.m. I would have to wait two hours to take my ten o'clock pills because calcium reduced the effect of Cyclo. With every meal, I drank a five ml dose of Nystatin. It prevented thrush, a common infection and a new risk being immuno-compromised.

At dinner I took more prednisone. Then eight p.m. cyclo and ten o'clock meds. When you are accustomed to taking pills for most of your life, shifting the routine is not difficult.

My new lungs were functioning well. My pulse-ox read ninety-nine to one hundred percent every time a nurse or respiratory therapist checked it. I could not remember ever scoring that well before. On Monday, I had to have a PICC line installed in my arm. PICC stands for peripherally inserted central catheter. It went in the arm and extended for eighteen inches. I would need it because once I got home, I would receive an antiviral drug called Gancyclovir for ten days. I also had Cytogam due every two weeks until June, and then once a month until August. They would both burn through normal veins so the catheter had to be placed in a larger one.

An IV tech came to install the PICC line. She looked just like Amy Kines back home and that made me relax a little. I got nervous about the PICC line, but she assured me that it would feel like any other IV. I could not watch, and kept my head tilted towards the window. In my mind, I started playing the Chequessett golf course on Cape Cod. I had played it so often every summer that I knew it backwards and forwards. I could smell the clean, salty air blowing off Wellfleet Harbor. I knelt down and felt the moisture on the green. I could see the Cape Cod sunlight washing against the scrub pines, and tall grass rustling at the mouth of the Herring River. I ended up scoring much better than in real life. I played the entire course a second time and a third.

The tech could not thread the catheter properly. It kept sticking on valves in my vein. Kristi Gott and Dr. Stang came by to talk while she worked.

For an hour and a half, she dug through my arm. Finally, I asked her to stop. It was clear that she was not making any progress and my nerves were shot. Normally, an IV tech tries three times to hit a vein. If they fail, they get someone else to try. My veins were very good, the result of years of weight lifting and ice hockey. People never had problems hitting my "ropes."

Desiree took care of me that afternoon and I asked her for something to help me relax. She brought me some Atavan and I dozed off.

Judy was concerned that the PICC line was not placed. She scheduled me in vascular radiology. They would place it using a fluoroscope. I was glad. Because of my kidney failure, I knew the folks who worked there and I trusted them.

Tuesday morning, Dr. Jones said that my chest tubes could be removed. That meant that I could go home a day later. Dr. Jones asked me what I wanted to do first thing when I got home. Actually, I had not really taken the time to think about it. After a moment, though, I knew: "I want to play with my dog, Bogart."

Dr. Ball came to my room along with Siobman, and Carrie. Carrie gave me a shot that contained six mgs of Demerol. I knew the removal would probably hurt. Dr. Ball asked me to climb into bed. That hurt a great deal because my tubes were so sore. They had now been in for sixteen days. I could barely lean back on my own.

Dr. Ball removed the dressings. He snipped the sutures that held the tubes in place, and he yanked the two tubes on my right side simultaneously, one in each hand. As he pulled, he told me to flex my diaphragm hard, as if going to the bathroom. I closed my eyes and tried to think about hockey. I heard a gurgling sound, like water draining out of a tub. It was very uncomfortable. As soon as he yanked the tubes out, Siobman covered each hole with a thick wad of gauze to stop the bleeding. She applied heavy pressure, leaning her body weight over me. While she did that, Dr. Ball sutured each hole shut very tight. That proved excruciatingly painful. My skin was very sore and he pulled the thread tight to seal the holes. I held on to Carrie's hand.

As he prepared to remove my two left tubes, I asked him to numb the area with Lidocaine. He looked a bit put out, but agreed. That helped a little, but it still hurt very badly. I wish I had been asleep for it.

After it was over, I felt immediate relief. Now I could inhale without pain. Now I could breathe much easier than before my transplant. Dr. Detterbeck and Dr. Jones came into my room soon afterwards and found me elated. I was up and about, and extended my arms to show them that I didn't have any tubes in me. For the first time in over two weeks, I wasn't connected to a wall suction unit or a machine. I was so happy that I gave them each a huge hug. Karen said it was one of the most moving moments she has ever witnessed.

They were privately worried that my lungs might collapse and kept a close eye on me for the rest of the day. I knew my lungs would be fine.

After Dr. Jones and Dr. Detterbeck left, Carrie took me on a field trip. We took an elevator downstairs and slipped out a back door. There I inhaled fresh air with new lungs for the first time. It tasted good.

Now that my chest tubes were out, I could work out down in physical therapy. Wednesday morning, I arrived in PT to find Mary Ellen and Michael Ackerman already there. Nanette came down a few minutes later. A number of family members were down in PT with them: Mary Ellen's husband, Gerald and her son, Daniel; Michael Ackerman's mother, Verna; and Nanette's dad, Mr. Yeomans. Mom and Karen had accompanied me.

I climbed onto the treadmill and began my workout. After twenty minutes, Carrie came down and told me that Vascular Radiology would be inserting my PICC line in a half an hour. She brought me some Atavan to help me relax. It would kick in right about when the procedure would begin.

I was upset that I could not work out in PT longer, but I did not want to miss my appointment in Vascular Radiology. They were very busy, and might not be able to reschedule me easily. Judy had told me that I would not be able to leave the hospital without a PICC line. So I was motivated.

Karen left to run errands and Mom took me to Vascular Radiology. We waited for a while, then were ushered in. It was the same team that placed my catheter for dialysis. The Atavan failed to relax me so I asked for some more stuff. They firmly believed in making patients comfortable, and gave me a shot of Demerol. They asked me to lie down on the table, and I needed help. My torso was very sore. The tech and I talked hockey. They numbed a site on the inside on my left bicep with Lidocaine. After that, I felt nothing. Soon, I had a very large catheter in my arm, extending eighteen inches into my body. It would last for a long time if need be.

After that, I walked back up to Anderson Four and Carrie removed the central IV line in my neck. Now I was cleared to go home. My chest tubes were out. My PICC line was in. I knew my new medicine schedule. Judy stopped by my room to go over everything. She realized that I still had not been taught how to give myself a shot of insulin. She told me I would have to stay another day to learn that. Then she stepped out to check something.

Carrie came in and I asked her to teach me how to inject insulin. Two and a half minutes later, I was fully educated. I never thought I would be able to give myself a shot, but when that stood between me and the door, I grabbed the syringe and inserted it.

When Judy returned a few minutes later, she was surprised that I was up to speed with my diabetes, but agreed that I could be discharged. I called Mom and asked her to come pick me up. Then Carrie helped me pack.

We were alone for a few minutes, and although I was not quite up for dating, I didn't want to blow my chances down the line. I also didn't want to make her uncomfortable by being hit on by a patient. So I put the ball in her court. I told her we should get together sometime, and gave her my number. That way, if she wanted to, we could go out.

At four o'clock, Carrie escorted Mom and me downstairs and out the front door of the hospital. It was April 30th, seventeen days after my operation. Together, Carrie and I waited as Mom got the car from the parking deck across the street. Finally when Mom came, I hugged Carrie goodbye, thanked her for everything and left.

My family was scared about bringing me home. It was like adopting a puppy for the first time. "How do we do take care of him?" Mom asked Dr. Paradowski. "He'll tell you what needs to be done," she replied.

The first thing I did when I got home was to take a scissors and snip the blue plastic hospital ID bracelet off my wrist. Freedom.

That night, Mom, Karen and I went out to dinner. I could go anywhere. What did I feel like eating? My family wrongly thought that I had digestive problems and had been subsisting on chicken broth and Jell-O. Actually, for the past week, my appetite was strong. That night, I wanted veal Parmesan, one of my all-time favorite foods. So we went to the Olive Garden.

When we arrived at the restaurant, we went a little bug crazy, extremely fearful of germs. The hostess offered us a table next to a large party of college kids. That would be no good. Next she offered us a table next to a family with small children. No thank you. Could we have a booth off in the corner, all alone? The hostess probably thought we were conducting a drug deal. But she found us a private table.

Normally, I would have started the meal with a salad. For the next three months, I would not be allowed to eat fresh fruit or vegetables. Since I wanted nutrition, I ordered a fried vegetable appetizer. After scarfing it down, I devoured the entire veal entree, a number of bread sticks, and pasta. Mom and Karen watched in amazement.

That night, I climbed into my own bed. I had been heavily reliant on the mechanized hospital bed, and reclining on my own was very painful. My voice was still totally shot, so if I needed any help, I could not be heard in the other rooms. I still had the terrible insomnia that had plagued me in the hospital. I did not fall asleep until after midnight, and woke up for the day at four a.m., Thursday.

When I awoke, I tried to adhere to every rule possible. My new morning routine should be done at the same time every day. I needed to check my vital signs: weight, temperature, blood pressure and pulse. I had to check my pulmonary function. Judy had given me a Datalog, my own PFT machine. It consisted of a mouthpiece connected to an analyzing computer and modem. I was supposed to blow into it three times. Everyday, it would automatically transmit my test results to a company in Minnesota, which in turn, would send the results to Judy.

That first morning, I faced a dilemma. I was supposed to check all of my vitals and PFTs as soon as I awoke. But I was also supposed to check them at the same time every day. It was four a.m. Surely, I would not be up every day at four. So I decided to wait until six.

Then I opened up my transplant logbook and recorded my first day's entry.

I set up my Datalog and blew into it. My FVC and FEV1 were the same: 1.55 liters. My FVC was less than before my operation, but my FEV1 was slightly higher. The numbers had never been the same before. When I spoke to Judy that morning, she was sure I had recorded my numbers incorrectly or not done the test properly. I assured her I had. It made no sense to her that the entire amount of air I blew out was the same amount that I exhaled in the first second. So she checked with Kristi. Kristi explained that it was common immediately post transplant for both numbers to be the same. Judy was new at this and still learning.

1.55 liters was not a huge amount of air to blow. It was barely a significant increase over my thirty percent lung function prior to transplant. But Ian had told me that it took months for the new lungs to fully inflate to their total capacity so I was not worried when I saw my numbers.

There were other rules I had to be aware of. Because of Aspergillus, I could not keep any plants in the apartment. And due to my compromised immune system, I was at a higher risk for skin cancer. If I went outside, I had to wear sun screen. Mom and Karen went out and bought me three different kinds that ranged from SPF 30 up to SPF 50. Every day, I diligently lathered up with the stuff. As a result, I smelled like the beach with a rich aroma of cocoa-butter wafting about.

Thursday, Bogart came home. Sherry had taken him to her apartment. She reported that like at Summit Hill, he became the neighborhood busybody, staring out the window all day at the comings and goings. One day, she left the blinds lowered thereby obstructing his view. The dog, in his enthusiasm, ripped them down. On another occasion, he helped himself to a chicken dinner that she left on the table. Even given all that, Sherry still doted on him. He had been a good playmate to Sherree, Sherry's granddaughter.

When Bogart came home, I was very happy to see him. He went nuts, scurrying from room to room, sniffing me, then Mom and Karen. He did not seem to notice anything different about me. In fact, he was indifferent.

On Thursday, I could remove the dressings that covered my chest tube sites. They were covered by a massive amount of surgical tape, thick, and strongly adhering to my skin and hair. Karen and I went into my bathroom, and I went through half a bottle of Detachol, scrubbing the tape and slowly peeling it back. I removed it all myself, and it hurt.

Even after all the tape was off, I still had to scrub adhesive muck that clung to me. Finally, it was all off and that felt great. I was one step closer to complete freedom.

That afternoon, two nurses from a home health company came to get me set up with Gancyclovir. I would infuse it once a day for the next week. One was training the other, who had just joined the company. I noticed almost immediately that the senior nurse had a cough. The last thing I needed was to catch a cold my first day out of the hospital. I asked her to put a mask on, but she did not want to. She explained that she had allergies. I did not believe her. So I asked her to leave. She did not want to leave. Then I asked the junior nurse to deal with the situation, which she did, and her partner donned a mask.

Thursday night, I dropped my bottle of insulin on the kitchen floor. The thin glass vial shattered. I freaked out. The local pharmacy had already closed, so I paged the lung transplant coordinator on call. Judy told me not to worry. They would probably switch my insulin around tomorrow at clinic.

Friday, I was still very sore. I was trying to wean my dose of Percacet down, fearful of frying my stomach. I spent the entire morning at the hospital. The first thing I had to do was get my blood drawn. Judy told me not to eat anything beforehand, so I arrived at the blood lab right when it opened, eight a.m. A line had already developed. I had brought my forms, but didn't know how to properly fill them out. Those lessons took place in an Atavan fog. Michael Ackerman was in the waiting area outside the blood lab, and he showed me what to write. He was very organized and had a supply of forms in a notebook.

The blood lab waiting room was jam packed with transplant patients. Because the picnic was the following day, many people scheduled their yearly clinic visit accordingly. It would be a long morning, but educational. I got to meet a number of people who were years out.

As I waited in the blood lab, I met Jeff. He lived in Alaska and worked as an outdoor electrician. Year round. His transplant had occurred four years ago and he looked great. He had a beautiful, supportive wife, and was clearly enjoying life. I asked him if he had any tips for ingesting Neoral, and he told me that the smell did not bother him.

After waiting forty-five minutes, I got my blood drawn and proceeded to x-ray. Michael was ahead of me and we waited together in the mens' dressing room. As we waited for the x-ray tech to call us, Michael started stretching. He twisted his torso to each side, and raised his arms high above his head. I gaped. Nobody had told me to start a stretching routine. Michael told me that when he was in the hospital, the therapists had gone over it with him. It prevented a loss of mobility. I got very upset at the thought of not doing absolutely everything by the book.

Like Tom Faraday, I could see Michael spreading his wings and becoming a new person. No longer was he dependent on oxygen. No longer did he need to conserve his energy. He was two weeks ahead of me in the recovery arc and bravely leading the way.

Michael proceeded on to physical therapy. I had to miss it because I had to go to clinic. First, I had to eat breakfast. That presented a problem. I did not want to take my mask off in the hospital. But I had to eat. I had brought a carry-out breakfast from Hardees, three bacon egg and cheese biscuits. Mom and I went outside to the picnic tables in an outdoor courtyard underneath the cafeteria. There I ate as she watched.

By nine-thirty, I was at transplant clinic. I waited for an hour. As I waited, I met a few more transplant recipients. I met Monica Goretski, who had for me been the epitome of smooth sailing. She still looked beautiful. We spoke for the first time. She told me that she lived in Mississippi and was studying to be a teacher.

Finally, I went into an exam room and met with Dr. Rivera and Judy. Dr. Rivera thought I looked good. Then I started asking questions that I had written down. What's the best way to bathe? Then I told her that I urinated excessively at night. My weight dropped six pounds from bedtime to wake up. I also had terrible night sweats, drenching my clothing and sheets as I slept. Dr. Rivera explained that it was probably from my elevated glucose. As my appetite increased, I wasn't taking in enough insulin. The high glucose acted as an "osmotic agent," making my body excrete fluid. Dr. Rivera also suggested that I might have a urinary tract infection. I would have to leave a urine sample, just to rule that possibility out. I had gone just before she made the request and had absolutely nothing to offer.

Again, I asked if we could plan a trip to Cape Cod for August. My three month mark would fall mid-July. At that point I would be allowed to move back to Maryland. Dr. Rivera explained that three month number was not set in stone, and they were not sure yet whether I could go to the Cape. Time was running out for us. The summer rentals usually sold out by late winter.

The last thing Dr. Rivera and I spoke about was my pain medicine. I had weaned myself down to two Percacets a day. She encouraged me to take as much as I needed and not hold back. It was important for me to be able to take deep breaths without pain.

The morning wore on and on. Finally, by 12:30, I was exhausted and hungry. They wanted me to stay in clinic but I just had enough. I wanted to eat lunch and take a nap. So I left.

Karen had lunch waiting for me when we got home. Organic, low-sodium vegetable soup. A low-sodium tuna sandwich. Low sodium potato chips. Canned pears. I ate it all and went to sleep. When I awoke, I needed some help getting up. I tried to call for Karen but she could not hear me. Then Bogart had a "Lassie" moment. He had been sleeping on the floor by my side, and when he heard me trying to get Karen, he got up and dragged her in. When I dozed off again, she proceeded to nap on the floor that afternoon so she could hear me if need be. After that, we kept a tin pot and a metal spoon by my bed. It wasn't quite a crystal bell, but it worked. It was loud.

That day, Bogart's demeanor changed completely. He would not leave my side all day. He followed me from room to room, hovering. It was really funny.

Late that afternoon, Dad arrived. He could not believe how good I looked. The last time he saw me, I still had four chest tubes. A considerable amount of tension melted off him.

∗∗∗

The next day was Saturday, May first. The picnic. Cousin Jonathan's parents, Lenore and Michael flew in from Dallas to be with us. They met us at the picnic.

The weather did not fully cooperate that day. A light drizzle misted the air. The picnic area had a covered roof with open sides, so the picnic proceeded. Michael and his mother came; Mary Ellen, her husband Gerald, and her son Daniel came. Nanette was still in the hospital, so she couldn't come. Ian wasn't there either. He had told me that he planned to be there. And Charity wasn't there. All in all, about twenty-five transplant recipients came. So did Melissa, who was still on the waiting list.

Everyone wore a name tag that included the date of their transplant. The recipients who were a few years out told me that at first, they diligently marked off monthly anniversaries. Now, though, they did not even think about when their operation took place.

My voice was non-existent, still aggravated from the ventilator. I wanted so badly to speak with everyone, and tried despite my laryngitis.

The food itself proved to be very depressing. I was hungry and loved picnic food. Annie Downs manned the buffet line. Will Crowder worked the grill. I picked up a plastic plate and surveyed the options. The hamburgers and hot dogs looked good, but then I realized that there was nothing else I could eat. The salads contained fresh fruits and vegetables, all uncooked. The pastas had fresh black pepper. The deserts were taboo due to my diabetes. And the chips were all high in sodium. This was not good. I was very disappointed.

Then cousins Lenore and Michael arrived. It was great to see them. Cousin Lenore reminds me of Barbara Streisand. She wears the same glasses and hair style and speaks with the same New York accent. Her accent has actually persisted despite the fact that she has lived in Texas for the past thirty-five years. Cousin Michael is an audiophile, a skilled wood craftsman, and a cardiologist. He was in heaven talking about the surgery and meeting Dr. Egan.

At one point, I almost ruined my chances with a beautiful pediatric physical therapist named Jennifer. We had danced the salsa and meringue together a few weeks before my transplant. With a small nose, corn-blue eyes, and slender hips, she reminded me of Karen's friend Julie. She came to the picnic and I was once again working my ball game. Dad came over to say hello. "You must be Cathy," he greeted her. "Dad, you're getting me in trouble here," I joked, trying to downplay the situation. "This is Jennifer." I tried not to blush and Jennifer laughed.

Kristi Gott came to the picnic with her husband. So did Jean Rae. Jean had just given birth to a daughter who she proudly presented to everyone. Judy also came for a short period of time. She brought a boyfriend. She was on call that day and her beeper buzzed constantly.

Towards the end of the picnic, Will asked everyone to line up for a group photo. Mary Ellen, true to her "wild woman" nickname, mooned the spectators. I felt bold, standing side by side with these people with whom I shared so much.

CHAPTER 15

Week Four

When Karen and I returned home after the picnic, I asked her to call Ian back in Maryland to see why he didn't attend. I had been looking forward to seeing him. I asked Karen to say upon his answering the phone: "where the hell were you today?" in a joking voice. Unfortunately, she said it seriously. Ian responded: "I'm the sickest I've ever been." Karen was furious at me for putting her in a very awkward situation. Ian had a terrible infection, a sepsis in his blood. It was caused by a home health nurse not handling an IV properly. He came down to UNC a few days later.

Saturday night, the family went out to a fancy Italian restaurant on Franklin Street. Once again, we went bug crazy. This time, we surpassed our performance in The Olive Garden. In retrospect, we may have gone a bit overboard just in ordering a glass of water for me.

The first time the waitress brought me a glass of water, it included a sliver of lemon rind. That was no good. It was a fresh fruit. So we sent it back.

Mom, Dad, Karen, and cousins Michael and Lenore each tried to educate the poor waitress. "He had a double lung transplant," explained one person. "His immune system is compromised" said another. "He can't have any raw fruit or vegetables," added a third. "None." "Zip." "Zilch."

Then she brought out a glass of sparkling water, which contained sodium. That went back. Finally, I got a glass of tap water. I was afraid to down it lest I require a refill.

That night, comedian Chris Rock caused me serious pain. We watched his HBO special and he forced me to laugh much harder than my body could withstand. For the rest of the summer, Karen and I walked around repeating a few memorable, but unprintable lines from his routine.

✳✳✳

That Sunday, I took my last Percocet pain killer. Since Friday, I had only taken two a day. I was sore, but no more so than on a higher dose. I could have remained on it longer, and still had half a bottle. I could have weaned down to Tylenol. But I decided stop all pain meds entirely and see how I felt. It was three weeks to the day after my operation.

✳✳✳

My diabetes got worse in the ensuing days. I began checking my glucose four times a day. Most of the time, it ran in the mid-two hundred range. Sometimes it went up into the three hundreds. Clearly, I was not taking in enough insulin, and I was not eating properly.

Insulin is measured in "units." Each unit represents one hundredth of a cc. The transplant team had me mixing two kinds of insulin, the "N" or long acting insulin, and "R" or medium length acting. I took a total of twenty four units a day in two shots. Judy knew that I needed more, but feared raising the dose too quickly.

Judy and I spoke almost daily. She was my lifeline to the transplant team. She controlled how I took care of myself and we became very close. Most mornings, she came down to PT to see us. By a random twist of fate, she was the transplant coordinator in charge of Michael, Mary Ellen, Nanette, and myself. As we worked out on the treadmills and stairmasters, she reviewed our logbooks, inspected our incisions, and answered our myriad questions. Every morning, I hoped she would come down. I liked seeing her, and I wanted her to be impressed by my progress on the machines.

Every few days or so, after reviewing my glucose record in my transplant log book, she raised my insulin by about two units. She did not want to raise it every day because each new dose of insulin needed a few days to balance out. If she gave me too much insulin, my glucose could crash. That would mean a very low blood sugar, less than seventy. So far, I seemed to be in little risk of that.

Although I knew I needed more insulin, I did not adjust my dose myself. A few years earlier, I had heard Dr. Egan make an offhand comment about that. Another patient had adjusted his own insulin dose, and Dr. Egan told him that he would end up in a box if he continued to do that. I kept that in mind.

Each time I checked my glucose, I pricked my finger and dabbed the blood on a tiny test strip. Then the glucometer would measure the glucose on the strip. It would take forty-five seconds to get a reading. As I waited, I crossed my fingers and said to myself, This is going to be good. It never was.

Despite giving myself more insulin, my glucose remained elevated. Some days were better than others, but my sugar almost never fell within the normal range of seventy to one hundred twenty.

I did not know this at the time, but high glucose is a serious matter. When glucose is elevated, it destroys the arteries and veins. The damage to the circulatory system causes blindness, nerve damage, renal failure, and loss of extremities. It also impedes the body's ability to heal.

***

On Monday, May fifth, I went to rehab for the first time as an out-patient after my transplant. Again, I first had to go to the blood lab on an empty stomach. It didn't open until eight. There was already a line, and I had to wait until almost nine o'clock. That was when PT began. So I had five minutes to go outside, eat a carry-out Hardees breakfast, and take my medicine. I felt as if my life had no leeway or margin for error.

Rehab was very gratifying. I focused incredibly hard on getting better. I put on a surgical mask before entering the hospital. I donned my workout shorts.

Mary Ellen, Nanette, Michael and I became very close at rehab. I suggested that we give our group a name. Michael coined the name "The Fighting Foursome," and we all liked it. Then we decided to give each other nicknames. Mary Ellen already had one: "Wild Woman." Michael thought up "little bit" for Nanette because each day, she was able to bike or walk just a little bit farther. Mary Ellen dubbed Michael "Superman" because he was so strong and fast on the treadmill. She called me "Roadrunner" because I tore it up on the stairmaster and treadmill. Each day, I climbed more and more flights. When I spoke to Mike Taylor on the phone, the first thing he would ask me was "how many flights did you climb today?"

During those initial weeks in rehab, we only had two choices that Angie played on the stereo: "The Blues Brothers Soundtrack" and "Disco Hits of the Seventies." Our old DJ/ tech had moved to New York and taken her vast music collection. Soon, we all got very bored with the Blues Brothers. So one day, Karen and I went to the mall and stocked up on CDs. I bought U2, Soul Hits of the Seventies; Heat Wave's Greatest

Hits; Kodo Japanese drumming; and Jane's Addiction. The Jane's Addiction CD included a song that we played first thing every morning to get us pumped up: "Been Caught Stealing." I needed to hear it played very loud. My litmus test was that people from other departments had to start complaining about the noise. That was when I knew it was at a sufficient decibel level.

On Monday, I asked Annie about stretching. She was horrified that none of the therapists had started me on a stretching program. She gave me a handout and went over it with me. I was to go through the program at least once a day.

We all worked up a sweat in rehab. The air was warm to begin with, so Angie hooked up small fans to the front of our machines. I would stare hard at the fan as I climbed and walked. I focused on it as I entered the zone.

Every day, we had a small audience as we worked out. A row of chairs backed up against the wall that faced us. There, our family members would watch us and we got to know each other. Nanette's dad, Mr. Yeomans came. So did Mary Ellen's husband Gerald, and her son, Daniel. Daniel would show off his new Jurassic Park wrist watch. Gerald would talk about fishing and golf. Michael's mother, Verna came. Karen and Mom took turns taking me.

In rehab, I wanted to work out my upper body, but could not because of the PICC line in my arm. Once that came out, then I could use the arm bike. I would not be able to lift weights for three months for fear of separating my sternum. Michael's was unstable and caused him discomfort. Ian had problems with his long after his operation. Charity's sternum hadn't settled down a year after her transplant. So I was content to wait.

***

When I returned home from the hospital, Karen devoted her life to taking care of me. She had never done so before because I had never needed it. But now, she helped me get dressed in the morning. I could not raise my arms above my head, so she helped me get my shirt on. Actually, I practically lived in my hockey jerseys. They were baggy which made them easy to get on and off without much mobility, and they had room in the arms for my PICC line.

Karen helped bathe me. My chest tube sites were still forming scabs. My incision had a small, one half centimeter opening at one end, under my left arm pit. That was normal, but I had to keep it protected. Because of those two factors, I could not shower. So I took sponge baths. The process began with Karen's ritual disinfecting of the entire bathroom. She sprayed the tub with anti-bacterial Lysol bathroom cleaner. She rinsed it off, and did the same to the sink and counter.

Karen went to Wal-Mart and bought a stack of ten wash cloths. We would go through the entire pile with one bath. She diligently scrubbed my body with anti-bacterial Palmolive. She rinsed and dried me off. She helped me get dressed. It would take forty-five minutes. Then she did a load of laundry for all of the washcloths.

Every day, Karen disinfected the entire apartment. She Lysoled the TV remote, the doorknobs and the lightswitches. She scrubbed down the kitchen and the dining room. She demonstrated initiative and zeal.

In the hospital, we used an instant hand sanitizer that consisted of foamed alcohol. Dispensers were mounted on most of the walls. When we got home, we tried to purchase a can, but because it was a hospital product not meant for consumers, we would have to buy a case for over $200. Mom started hunting around for a comparable product. Finally, at Bath and Body Works, she found a scented alcohol gel that was essentially the same thing. A few months later, we found an even better product, Purell, at our local supermarket. It did not contain perfume.

Some people feel that it is foolish to go to such an antibacterial extreme. They say that you need to expose yourself to the everyday germs out there so that your body can build up an immunity to them. In those first few months after transplant, however, we did not want to take any chances.

We began to live an existence not unlike one described my Michael Crichton in his novel, *The Andromeda Strain*. The book is about a group of government scientists who try to determine the cause of death of an entire town. They suspect that a deady virus arrived on an errant meteor. To test their hypothesis, they go to a facility specifically designed to safely handle biohazards. The building is underground and contains five levels, each one more clean than the one above it. To pass to another level, the scientists must decontaminate themselves even more. They wear paper clothing that is incinerated at each juncture. They get sprayed. And they get thoroughly cleansed to the point where they must get naked and swim completely underwater through disinfectant to pass to the next level.

At this point, I also began to see the world through eyes portrayed in the movie *Basic Instinct*. Early on, detectives investigate the scene of a terrible murder. They spray the scene with a product called Luminol and then shine a black light. All body fluids become illuminated. They appear like globs on the walls, furniture and carpeting. I began to see purple blotches of imaginary bacteria on the walls, floor, and counters.

Handling money was a concern. As it passes from hand to hand, it becomes very dirty. I washed my hands very frequently, probably to the point of obsessive/ compulsive disorder.

We began to keep a separate stick of margarine in the refrigerator for me. That was because people used their own knives instead of a butter knife, and we felt that germs might get passed along.

✳✳✳

The great fallacy of smooth sailing is that there is such thing. Even people who do well after transplant have their share of problems. It is just a matter of degrees. While I continued to progress, I still had my bumps.

By the end of that first whole week home, my weight had plummeted twenty pounds. I still lost six pounds every night from terrible night sweats and excessive urinating. That water weight was very difficult to replace during the day. Judy asked me to check my temperature and glucose when I was up in the middle of the night. Testing my blood was difficult enough four times a day. Five was very hard. But I did it. Each night, my glucose ran in the mid to high two hundreds. No wonder I lost so much weight.

I had other minor problems. My legs swelled during the day. The first time I noticed it, I was shocked. My legs looked huge and my feet felt as if a load of jelly sat atop them. Angie explained that leg swelling was normal after surgery. I should try to sleep with my legs elevated. That helped and each morning, my legs would be normal. Cousin Michael told me to be careful because that edema could bruise very easily. He said the swelling might continue for up to six months. Other minor inconveniences included an eye twitch; a runny nose; and a slight loss of balance.

***

Rehab was scheduled for Monday, Tuesday, Wednesday and Friday mornings. Thursday we had off. At least three days a week, Judy had me check my blood. My Cyclosporin level in my blood was very low. She kept raising the dose, but it failed to rise. Getting the dose right is a tricky business. If it is too low, then the patient is not protected from rejecting the new organ. If it is too high, kidney damage can result. Because CF is a digestive disease, the Cyclosporin level is directly affected by how well we happen to be absorbing our food on a given day. This meant that until we got my dose correct, I had to have my blood checked very often.

During week four, I decided that it would be easier to come in on Thursday to have my blood tests and x-rays done than to try to squeeze them in before rehab on another day.

At the end Tom Wolfe's novel, *The Bonfire of the Vanities,* Sherman McCoy is relegated to a life fighting the criminal court system in New York. Consequently, he gets to know how to dress for jail, with khakis and hiking boots. That is exactly how I felt, only with the hospital. Each morning before rehab, I would pack up a small bag with what I would need for my excursion into the depths of the healthcare system. I would pack a face mask; my log book; completed forms for the blood lab and x-ray; two bottles of water; a can of Caffeine Free Diet Coke to drink with my Cyclosporin; breakfast from Hardees; alcohol; insulin; handi-wipes; and my ten o'clock meds. I would wear sweat pants and jogging shorts underneath.

Friday, I had my first six-minute walk after my transplant. Angie tethered me up to a pulse-ox and off we went. Karen tagged along. During that walk, I set a UNC transplant record. I became the first person to run four weeks after his operation. During the test, I actually sprinted. Angie could not believe it. I wanted to run very badly, and for the first few steps down the hospital corridor, my legs felt like rubber. I thought they might collapse underneath me. But I pushed past the rubbery feeling and I could feel them strengthen beneath me. Angie and Karen both struggled to keep up with me. In the end, I was out of breath and totally spent, leaning against the wall for dear life.

In six minutes, I ran 2,126 feet, just seventy-five feet shy of my last walk before transplant. Annie Downs explained to me that the amount of distance people lose in that time frame varies by the condition they are in before transplant. Losing seventy-five feet meant that I was in very good shape.

I was so happy about sprinting that I told everyone about it for the rest of the day. In the afternoon, Mom told a friend of hers on the phone: "He went jogging this morning." Wrong. I had to correct her on the spot.

"I was sprinting, not jogging."

***

Because of my persistent high glucose, Judy scheduled me to meet with Emily Brimseth, the team nutritionist. Emily met me in rehab and took me down to her office. She gave me advice about how to eat properly with Diabetes. I should try to eat meals at the same time every day. I should eat green vegetables with lunch and dinner. That would help me breakdown glucose. I should eat the same amount of calories in each meal, and I should eat the same amount of protein, carbohydrate and fat with each meal. Say what? I had no idea how on Earth to accomplish that. She asked me to keep a diary of my food intake and we would go over it together. She analyzed my meals and said they were very inconsistent. They were also very high in fat and sodium. The Hardees bacon, egg and cheese biscuits were not helping. I did not know what to do. I had to eat outside after blood and before PT. Hardees was located right next to Summit Hill. Other food choices between my apartment and the hospital were scant. Emily suggested substituting an orange for a biscuit. That would help. "Doesn't that violate the no fresh fruit rule?" I asked, very frustrated. Emily explained that if Mom or Karen totally disinfected the skin and then peeled it for me, an orange would be fine. Again, I felt as if I had no margin for error. And I wondered how on Earth I could cram an orange into my already-full bag.

CHAPTER 16

Week Five

Monday, I received my second infusion of CytoGam. Linda McIlveen, a nurse from the home IV company, came to administer the dose. We hung out and talked for the entire two hour infusion. She asked me if I would go through the transplant again if I had to. After giving it some thought, I said that I probably would. All in all, it was not a situation I wanted to contemplate.

The last time I received CytoGam was the day I hung out with Dr. Yankaskis. I had not given it a second thought since. Then Mom, Karen and I went out to dinner with Sema Lederman. I ordered a steak and ate a few slices of bread. I didn't make it to the salad course. I ran off to the men's room, wrecking every chance I had at impressing this fine young woman. Karen drove me home and on the way we paged the lung transplant coordinator on call. It was Kristi's night. She told me that I should keep an eye on the situation. She didn't know what caused my nausea. I asked if I could take some Phenergan and she consented. Judy had

pounded into my head how important it was to check with the team
before taking any non routine medicine.

Phenergan offered me some relief and I soon dozed off. When I
awoke, Linda was over at the apartment checking on me. It was ten
o'clock at night. She told me that the CytoGam probably caused my
nausea. It was unusual, but likely.

By the end of my fifth week post-transplant, my PFTs had almost
doubled. My FVC was now 2.85 and my FEV1 was 2.55. I could not
remember the last time my FEV1 was that good. I was learning how to
get the optimum results on the PFTs. I found that if I blew each of the
three blows in immediate succession, they were not as good. If I rested
for ten minutes between blows, however, then they were much stronger.

✳✳✳

That Saturday, we went to synagogue. We found a conservative con-
gregation in Durham, just off of Duke's East Campus. A Bat Mitzvah
was in progress, so we slipped in the back. The sanctuary was packed
and we had trouble finding four seats. Because it was so crowded, I put
a mask on. An immuno-compromised existence was still new to me and
crowded public places made me nervous. People glanced over at us,
then refocused their attention on the rabbi and the young woman at the
center of the ceremony.

I felt that it was important to say thank you to God for providing me
with new lungs and getting me healthy again. I am not an especially religious person, but I knew that an expression of gratitude was important.
Some people go through transplant and because the process itself is
such a miracle, redouble their religious fervor.

✳✳✳

We made no progress in treating my diabetes. At the beginning of the
week, I took thirty three units of insulin a day. By the end, we raised it

to forty two. Even so, my glucose raged well into the three hundreds. This was very frustrating. Twice that week, Karen noticed a maple syrup smell emanating from me. I asked Judy if she were conferring with the doctors about my insulin dose. She got mad at me for not trusting her ability to manage my diabetes, but then admitted that she was in fact checking with Dr. Rivera. As Ronald Reagan would say, trust but verify.

In rehab, I began to suffer terrible leg cramps, mainly in my shins. The Prednisone had begun to chew up my muscles. I was taking sixty milligrams a day. After each workout, I would collapse onto a chair, nearly in tears. Angie would put ice packs on my legs to alleviate the pain.

My insomnia slowly abated over the ensuing weeks. For a while, I could sleep five hours a night, then six. Usually, after rehab, I would need a nap, and again, another one in the early afternoon. So I was beginning to get some serious rest.

***

Cyclosporin became more of a problem. The transplant team had a difficult time finding the right dose of Neoral for me. My levels kept coming back from the lab either too low or too high.

At first, Judy put me on a drug called Nizoral. When taken with Cyclosporin, it bumps up the effectiveness. Nizoral helped, but not enough. Nizoral was contraindicated with my antacid, Zantac, which I switched to Prilosec. It was also contraindicated with a laxative I took, Cisipride, which prevented bowel blockage. I could not replace Cisipride with a different brand and was terrified that with the high doses of calcium that I took to prevent further osteoporosis, I would block up. Luckily, I survived just fine without Cisipride.

Finally to regulate my Cyclosporin, Judy asked me to come in and have my blood drawn every hour for three hours after my dose. That way, they could track exactly how my body absorbed it.

As I sat there between blood draws, I met Kelly Helms. She had received a transplant five years earlier. Kelly was in her mid-thirties, lived in Florida, and worked for a large banking corporation. She competed in swimming and looked very healthy. We struck up a conversation. She told me how rough bronchoscopies used to be. In the past, the doctors did not believe in sedation and would conduct the procedure while patients were wide awake. She said it was so bad that her entire body would arch off the table. She and all of the other patients revolted. They refused to undergo bronchs anymore unless they were given anesthesia. The team consented. I had her to thank for the relative ease of my bronchs.

When the results of my timed cyclo levels came back, the team decided to put me on the drug three times a day, not just two. That was not fun. I still hated taking Neoral, and my stomach would still reflexively try to regurgitate each pill.

Slowly, over the next few weeks, I would become enured. At first, my stomach stopped shuddering. Then after a while, I realized that I did not need grape juice or Caffeine Free Diet Coke to help swallow each pill. I could use water. After that, it became easier and easier.

A few months later, I asked Judy if she could tell me the side effects of Cyclosporin. She e-mailed me the following list: "reduction in short-term memory, hypertension, hirsuitism, tremors, gingival hypertrophy (swelling of the gums), headaches, seizures, acne and leg cramps."

***

One month to the day after my transplant, I went on my first date. Cathy came over to see me. Karen and I went out to the parking lot to greet her. A lavender twilight stretched across the sky. Cathy squealed in delight upon seeing me. She wanted to check out my scar right away, in the parking lot. I lifted my shirt so she could see it. "Cool," she said.

We brought Cathy inside to meet Mom, and then Bill, a neighbor from upstairs, dropped by. We all ended up hanging out in the apartment, talking for a few hours. After Cathy left, Bill inquired about her. I told him to forget it. He got the picture.

The subject of dating caused great concern for Karen and she became very overprotective. Since I was immuno-compromised, Karen feared that every woman I went out with might be a breeding ground for infections. She did not want me to kiss anyone, much less have sex. She felt that I should "wrap myself in a full-body condom." I told Karen that if people couldn't have sex after their transplants, nobody would sign up for them. To be safe, I checked with Judy as to what I should keep in mind. She told me to practice "safe sex" and I would be fine. She also said that if my girlfriend or I had any specific questions, we could call her anytime.

That week, I returned to my computer. I checked my e-mail for the first time. My mail box had overflowed with over one hundred messages. I opened up my word processor and began recording my thoughts about my transplant. I knew I would otherwise forget my early experiences in the ICU and Anderson Four.

On Wednesday, we got a free lunch at Applebees. I think that was the highlight of the summer for Mom. The waiter failed to deliver our lunch in fourteen minutes, as guaranteed. Mom got very excited. Halfway through my lunch, I looked down at my french fries and noticed black specks on them. I called the waiter over. "What are those specks?" I asked. "Fresh pepper," he replied. Of course, we had gone through our entire spiel about no fresh fruit or vegetables, and no black pepper. Regardless, my hamburger arrived with fresh lettuce and tomato garnishing the plate, my water had a lemon wedge, and the fries had pepper. That happened at almost every restaurant we patronized.

Mom and Karen freaked out when they learned that I had just eaten half an order of fries with black pepper. They were convinced that I would contract Aspergillus. I was relaxed about it. There was nothing I could do about it now, so why worry? "Should we page Judy?" Karen asked. "No."

One day, Karen and I were hanging out in the living room, watching TV. By chance, she opened up the closet and I caught a glimpse of my ThAirapy Vest and nebulizer. I had not seen either machine since April 12th. I realized that I had not needed five hours a day of respiratory therapy since then. I had not needed any. It was wonderful. My new lungs did not have CF and never would. CF is genetic, and the cells in my donor lungs were not encoded with that faulty programming.

***

Karen was scheduled to go back to Boston on Friday. But Thursday night, my incision opened up three quarters of an inch. No big deal. It didn't hurt at all. I only noticed it in the bathroom mirror when I brushed my teeth. The incision had opened up before but this time Karen got very upset. Mary Ellen had endured a major, four inch opening the prior week that had required a visit to the emergency room, packing and stitches. I knew mine did not merit that. We paged the lung transplant coordinator on call. Again, it was Kristi. I'm sure that I woke her up. Kristi asked us to describe the opening. She asked what type of bandages and antiseptic supplies we had in the house. We were fully stocked. "All of the above," I told her. She said to clean the opening thoroughly and then place a steri-strip across it. Judy could check it the next day in clinic.

It was twelve thirty at night. After "nurse" Karen diligently did everything that Kristi prescribed, she went back into her room and I went to bed. As I lay there in the dark, I heard her on the phone with US Airways, changing her plane reservation from Friday to Saturday. She did not want to leave because of my incision. I thought that was nice, but completely unnecessary.

That Saturday, Karen did leave. It was sad, but she and Mom had not been getting along well. I was caught in the middle constantly, but because my voice had not yet returned, I could not get a word in edgewise. I suggested that they rotate, Karen could go back to Boston for a few weeks, then she could return and Mom could go back to Maryland for a few weeks. They both liked that idea.

By now, I could put a shirt on by myself. I could bathe myself. I could cook for myself. I needed much less help navigating through life.

***

On Saturday, Cathy and I went out just the two of us. We went to an outdoor café. It overflowed with people from Duke celebrating graduation. The sun was out, and the temperature was warm. We sat at a table wearing sunglasses, sipping iced tea and looking very cool. We still had no major spark, but I liked being with her.

***

On Monday, I had my one month bronchoscopy. It was the second one of my life. Judy warned me that because I did not have all of the morphine swirling around inside me like I did for the first one, I might not be as sedated. I ended up waking up in the middle. I forced myself to keep my eyes shut because I did not want to see what was going on. I was uncomfortable but not in pain. I immediately began making an injection motion with my right hand toward my left forearm, like a heroin junkie. I wanted some more good stuff as soon as possible. Judy hollered at me to stop moving. She was giving me more medicine. Then I went right back to sleep.

We had a big problem when I awoke in the recovery room. Mom and I were sitting in big lounge chairs when a nurse approached us. She gently suggested that I move a few feet away from another patient. An elderly lady three feet away from me had tested positive for Tuberculosis.

They did not know whether or not the infection was active. She did not wear a mask. I did not want to take any chances with TB so I got dressed and walked out of recovery. The nurse tried to stop me. "A doctor needs to check you out." I was not about to wait for a doctor. So Mom and I walked up to the transplant office. A doctor could meet me there.

Judy got mad at us for leaving recovery. She felt that the day-op nurses would not endanger us. But Dr. Stang met us in the transplant office and agreed that we were right to leave. Mom was furious that the hospital would take such a risk with me or any of the other immuno-compromised patients.

I recovered quickly from my bronch. The next day at rehab, I resumed my progress without missing a beat. I climbed 31 flights on the Stairmaster. My strength was starting to really come back. I began twice-a-day workouts. In the afternoon, I would try to walk for a mile or so. One afternoon, the weather was especially beautiful so Mom and I went for a two and a half mile hike in Duke Forest. On the way home, we stopped by Eckerd pharmacy to pick up a refill. There I bumped into Betty, the nursing assistant from Anderson Four. Seeing her just about made my week.

My only problem after the bronch was an occasional streak of blood in my spit. That is entirely normal. During a bronch, they remove eight to eleven tissue samples from the lungs. There is tearing, and a small amount of bleeding.

Michael and Mary Ellen had endured less positive bronchoscopies. Michael felt exhausted and out of sorts for a few days after his. During her first bronch after surgery, Mary Ellen suffered an internal bruise. A tech dropped the fluoroscope directly on her fragile sternum in the middle of the procedure. Clearly, there were serious risks and bronchs should not be taken lightly. I was very grateful that mine went as smoothly as they did.

On Friday, we had clinic and raised the TB issue with Dr. Rivera. She fully agreed that it was an outrage. "What could we do to prevent this from happening next time?" we asked her. Dr. Rivera promised to raise the issue with the other transplant doctors. That afternoon, she called us back at the apartment. She suggested that we write a letter and send it to the hospital brass. Then she gave us a list of people who should receive it.

That morning in clinic, Dr. Egan gave us the go-ahead for Cape Cod later in August. Dad called up real estate agents in Wellfleet that afternoon.

That weekend, Cathy and I went out again. Her mom was in town, visiting from Iowa. Bill came along and we went out to the movies. Then we went out for ice cream and sodas at Ben & Jerry's on Franklin Street.

***

Finally, I had time to watch the video that cousin Jonathan had given me in the hospital. It was hysterical, but not by intent. Cousin Jonathan is normally extremely animated and funny. He talks in a rapid fire streak, and a listener must pay close attention or miss out. I popped the video into my rented VCR and an entirely different person appeared on the screen. Not Cousin Jonathan, borscht belt comedian. This was cousin Jonathan, American gothic eulogist. His smile was gone. His demeanor serious. His speech slow and calculated. He sat in a rocking chair and read a passage from a book written by a business guru. The topic he read about proclaimed "You are the problem." It was very funny. I joked with him later on: was he trying to send me a not-so-subtle message?

***

My diabetes was now officially driving me crazy. I took sixty-four units of insulin a day, yet my glucose continued to spike into the three hundreds. Judy suspected that I developed a resistance to insulin. This is common with CF patients. By the end of the week, I was up to seventy four units of insulin, with no progress at lowering my blood sugar.

On Monday, I had another dose of CytoGam. I was very nervous about getting nauseous again. Linda McIlveen had checked with the home health pharmacist and they thought that if they ran the dose in slowly, over four hours instead of two, I might not have a reaction. They turned out to be right. I almost got nauseous, to the point where tiny jets of saliva spurted in my mouth, but it never progressed beyond that. A few hours later, I ate three burritos.

The following morning, I climbed one hundred and seven flights on the Stairmaster in thirty minutes. It was far more than I could do before transplant.

We had a new transplant recipient at rehab that week. Lil Schumaker received her new lung in the middle of the month. Seeing her was like looking into a reflection of who we were just one month earlier. Her arms were badly bruised from the numerous IVs and arterial lines. Our bruises were now healing. She walked slowly as her strength had not yet returned. And her spirits seemed modulated. Ours were starting to brighten.

We inducted Lil into our group and changed the "Fighting Foursome" to the "Fighting Fivesome" to accommodate her. We wasted no time in giving her a nickname: Flash. She earned that in the ICU, where, because of the heat and her cataracts, she wore no clothing, only sunglasses.

Wednesday night, Michael, Mary Ellen and I spoke at support group. We wanted to make a grand entrance so we arrived wearing "Blues Brothers" sunglasses. Nobody noticed. So much for going "Hollywood." We each described our transplant experience, soup to nuts. Now we took on the role that Ian had played before our operations.

Thursday night, I drove a car for the first time. Judy had instructed me not to drive until the following week. Dr. Rivera explained that they wanted me to be able to jerk a steering wheel without pain if I had to avoid hitting a squirrel. I could do that but Judy is very conservative by nature and wanted me to wait anyway. That Thursday, Mom and I went out for Greek food. I especially liked the restaurant because they offered thoroughly cooked vegetables. Afterward, Mom was sleepy, and I felt it was safer for me to drive than her. I still give her a hard time about that.

Back in Maryland, another dinner took place that same night. Mike Taylor, Mike Copperman, Mike Simpson, Jon Lastuvka and J.T. Jacoby took Dad out to dinner at Houston's, a popular hangout in Bethesda. They wanted to hear all about the transplant and how I was doing. Dad filled them in. Then for some unfortunate reason, they felt it incumbent upon themselves to fill him in on all of the great parties I had thrown in high school when my parents were out of town. Up until that point, they had been blissfully unaware.

To reciprocate, Dad described for them all of the women in North Carolina who kept coming over to visit me and who kept calling. That made a very big impression. The next morning, each one of them privately called to ask for the name of the movie that I saw with Annette and Jay just after I moved down. The one that I had recommended so strongly. The one that had apparently made such a big impact on my social life. The one that they never got around to seeing. After some persuasion, I told them once again: *Swingers.*

That morning, I walked Bogart alone for the first time. This was no small accomplishment. Inside the house, he is a sweet little angel. Outside, he becomes Mr. Hyde. His seventy pound body explodes with ferocity at any perceived threat, be it foreign or domestic. One must hold on tight to the leash and not be afraid of suffering a dislocated shoulder. I did not want to walk him until the doctors felt it was safe. Finally, they gave the okay.

Friday, I drove myself to rehab for the first time. By now, our audience had thinned a little. Michael's mother no longer came. Mom had taken to dropping me off and then going to hunt down a copy of the *New York Times* on Franklin Street. Gerald and Daniel came sometimes, but not always. Mr. Yeomans, Nanette's dad, always came, without fail. We could see how happy he was that his daughter was recovering so well. He smiled in constant contentment.

✳✳✳

Towards the end of the week, I called Carrie, my nurse from Anderson Four. Ever since I left the hospital, my family encouraged me to do so. I wanted to wait until I started to look good again, and finally felt near that point. I had gained back half the weight I lost and now weighed one hundred and forty pounds. So I left a message on her answering machine. She called back a month later. She did not want to go out. That really surprised my family. I think that like Judy, Carrie felt uncomfortable crossing the line that divides care giver and patient.

CHAPTER 17

Month Two

My PFT's did not change significantly from mid-May to the beginning of June. Ian had told me that my numbers would increase in plateaus. I was eager for them to improve but breathing well and happy about that.

I still had minor soreness, and some numbness along my incision. My chest tube scabs had looked pretty grizzly, but were now starting to peel off.

On Monday, I hit a personal record in rehab: one hundred and sixteen flights on the Stairmaster. Then I walked for thirty minutes at an eight percent grade on the treadmill. It was a tough workout, but I was very proud.

I decided that it was time to contribute a poster to rehab. It would have to be really good. I wanted future classes of transplant recipients to look at my poster and be motivated, just as I had been by those left by my predecessors. Subaru had run a print ad in the early eighties that I thought captured the spirit of what I wanted to convey. The headline read: "Before you can ski through the powder, you've got to pay your dues in the mud." I wrote a letter to the president of Subaru of America, Inc. asking for a copy of that ad.

***

Tuesday night, I went back to the Raleigh IcePlex and saw my old team play for the first time since my operation. The night after my transplant, April 14, The Pirates won the league championship. In lieu of trophies, we got t-shirts. Our captain presented me with mine when I arrived at the rink. At one point during the second period, my team-mate Mike Bowling pulled a Babe Ruth maneuver. Mike was a CAT scan tech over at Duke Medical Center. He was six feet four and well over two hundred pounds, a gentle giant off the ice. But on the ice, he was fierce. Midway during the second period, Mike pointed at me, then at the goal. Sure enough, he rocked one in for me. I pounded on the plexiglass with joy. My voice had just begun to come back and now I could cheer for the team. Mike went on to infamy, earning an ejection in the third period for fighting.

It was incredibly difficult to watch my friends play and not partici-pate. I wanted so badly to hit the ice, to experience what it felt like to play with new lungs. I deliberately left my gear at home because if it was in the car, the temptation would have been too great. Mom told me to relax. "I don't know how to repair sternums."

Mom liked Carolina for the most part. We went to see a play at NC State over in Raleigh. We toured an Art Museum, scoured the malls, and explored many of the dining opportunities.

Mom had one big problem with the state: the wildlife that invaded our apartment. Centipedes and ladybugs cohabitated with us at Summit Hill. They drove her crazy. She would patrol the apartment with a wad of newspaper, swatting away when she spotted them. She chastised Bogart for not scaring them off. When the weather heated up, the problem got worse. A five inch lizard moved into the patio area outside. It never came inside, but enjoyed sunning itself on the warm cement. Mom shrieked whenever she saw it, thereby terrifying the dog.

At least once a week, Mom called poor Beau over in the Summit Hill maintenance office and asked them to arrange another round of extermination for the centipedes and ladybugs. Beau would send over his extermination expert, a character not far off from John Goodman's fine model in "Arachnaphobia." Like Goodman's character, he mistakenly believed that "there are no spiders here." On one memorable day, the temperature ran up to about ninety-five degrees. That afternoon, our exterminator told us that "the critters would all go away once it got warm outside." This did not assuage Mom's concerns.

***

On Wednesday, Judy added a third shot of insulin to my routine. I did not look forward to three shots a day, but knew that my glucose was out of control. For the rest of the week, my numbers got better, never reaching as high as three hundred. They still went well into the two hundreds, but on three occasions out of twenty-eight, they were actually within the normal range of seventy to one hundred twenty. That was the best it had been since I began tracking it.

As soon as we added the third shot of insulin, my body weight responded. I urinated and sweated much less at night. My weight rose to one hundred and forty-eight pounds by Sunday night. My body spoke.

***

1997 set a record at UNC for the number of lung transplants. In June, we added two new recipients to rehab: Steve Roebuck and Queen Emerson. It was great to see Steve and Queen. We had followed their progress closely, from when they got their new lungs, to graduating from the ICU to Anderson Four, to their discharge from the Hospital. I knew Queen from support group. Like me, she had attended it through the winter and spring. Steve I did not know. He flew up to UNC from Georgia right when he got beeped. Like me, the ventilator did a number on his voice. I assured him that it would clear up. I told him that mine took six weeks to return to normal.

With seven of us, rehab got crowded and we had to coordinate our workouts carefully. Who wanted to use the bikes first and then the treadmill? Who wanted the armbike and the Stairmaster? In addition to Angie, there were two techs to help out.

***

One day, we received a phone call at the apartment. Jesse Helms, the senior Senator from North Carolina, wanted to congratulate me on becoming a North Carolina success story. Mom answered the phone and thanked him for the superb care I received at UNC Memorial Hospital. Then she handed me the receiver. All he wanted to talk about with me was my "vivacious momma." It was great. I recalled to him how he had given Karen and me a tour of the floor of the Senate when we were kids, and how we had both served as pages. He then promised to take us all to lunch when we returned to Washington.

***

I began to notice an excessive amount of hair sprouting out all over me. My arms had new blotches growing on my inner forearms. My ears had strands spiking off my lobes and out of my hearing canal. I felt like "Teen Wolf," the character in the Michael J. Fox movie.

On Thursday, Prednisone continued to wreak havoc on my muscles. As I ground away on the Stairmaster, my lower back developed serious pain. Not only did I fail to improve and do more, but my stamina regressed. Somehow I completed one hundred and five flights, but I could not handle any grade on the treadmill. I feared that a weak workout would hinder the inflation of my lungs. Mary Ellen cheered me up by showing off her electric blue panties as if she were a Moulin Rouge dancer. I reciprocated with my Stars and Stripes boxer shorts.

Prednisone offered me one completely bizarre and unexpected side effect. One morning, I called Judy and asked her if the drug could be making my nipples grow bigger. She said yes. Then I asked if that was the weirdest question I had yet put forth to her. She actually did not think so. After I mustered up the confidence to ask her about my nipples, they never looked big again. If only I waited a day. But the transplant team always said that if we weren't sure about something, we should call them.

I began to notice one other side effect, Cushingoid. Prednisone caused my cheeks to puff up. Mine was not too bad. Some of my friends' faces puffed up so badly that they were unrecognizable. It takes about a year or two for one's appearance to return to its former state.

***

That afternoon, Karen returned to Chapel Hill and Mom headed back to Bethesda. The Monday after she arrived, I had my last bi-weekly dose of CytoGam. It was seven weeks post transplant. After that, CytoGam would be administered once a month, and in half the strength. It meant that my PICC line could be removed. Susan, the nurse who treated me my first day after I got home, came over to take care of me.

As the medicine infused, we talked all about her main hobby, country-western dancing. Karen got all excited. She wanted to go. Ever since she began visiting me in Chapel Hill the prior Thanksgiving, I would catch her mumbling country music lyrics to herself as she puttered around the apartment. Most memorable was the Trace Adkins song "I left something turned on at home." Every time I got in my car after she had driven it somewhere, the radio had been tuned to a country music station. She had secretly been amassing a collection of country music

CDs. Susan invited us to go with her to the most famous club, The Longbranch. She was in her mid-forties and had a college aged-son, but was very sexy. I flirted with her and she flirted back. Then she admitted that she couldn't date patients. I held up my hand and said: "Stop the infusion," implying that then I would no longer be her patient. We all laughed.

When she removed my PICC line, I was finally free of all attachments. My body was a self-contained unit once again. That felt incredible. I only had a bandage to protect the PICC line site for two days. Then complete and utter freedom for the first time since that Sunday in April. I could now shower and not seal my arm in Saran wrap. I could now work out on the arm bike in rehab to build up my upper body strength.

On Thursday, my day off from rehab, I returned to the YMCA for the first time. I was a little nervous about walking through the locker room with such a huge scar from one armpit to the other. But I wanted to swim. That would help build up my strength. As I scrubbed in the shower, a few guys came in. One looked just like cousin Jonathan and had the same sense of humor. He took one look at my chest and made an admiring comment about my lines. He was impressed. I smiled and thanked him. After that, I didn't care who saw me. I strode out to the pool as if having those scars was the only way to be.

As I headed down the breeze way between the locker room and the pool, I realized that the only thing I carried was my beach towel. I did not bring a gym bag with a box of Kleenex. I subconsciously knew that I would not cough and need to spit during the workout.

I cannot deny the fact that a few jaws dropped when I arrived at the pool. Kids gaped. The lifeguard tried not to notice anything different. But I didn't care. I wanted to know what it would be like to swim with new lungs. I slowly inched my way into the water. The temperature was much cooler than it had been the last time I was there. I hate cold water, but somehow, I got in. Then I started swimming. No coughing. I was not out of breath. Now, my legs and arms lacked the strength I needed. I managed three laps, but knew that as my strength returned, I would be able to swim much further. I do not think it a coincidence that my PFTs bumped out of their plateau the week I hit the pool. Now my FVC was over 3 liters.

***

A week after switching to three shots of insulin a day, my glucose lapsed back into the terrible range of three to four hundred. At this point, Judy decided to refer me to the endocrinology clinic. She made an appointment for me for the following week.

"Endo" clinic was held in the ACC. It was very busy and I had to wait. Finally, I met with Dr. Buse and his team nutritionist, Elizabeth Bruntlett. Dr. Buse had a thick red beard and a beeper that rang even more often than Judy's. He had a stellar reputation and people sought his advice from far and wide. Elizabeth had a very slim waist; perfect posture; dark eyes that could easily have peered out from a middle eastern Chador; and a deep sense of composure. She looked formal and proper, but in conversation, she was very easy going and open. She dressed more upscale than most of the other people in the ACC.

Dr. Buse explained to me that both Prednisone and Neoral were probably causing my diabetes. I had thought it was just the Prednisone, but he explained that Cyclosporin had a similar effect. He said that I probably was resistant to insulin. Then he recommended I try carbohydrate counting. I would look at the food I was about to eat, count the amount of carbohydrates in the meal, and give myself a shot of Humalog insulin. He called it "rocket fuel" because it began working within ten minutes. I asked him a number of questions. Most importantly, I wanted to know if my diabetes would go away when the transplant team lowered my immuno-suppression doses at the six-month mark, November. A number of my friends had been insulin-dependent until that point, then gone off it. Dr. Buse said that it was a possibility. I also wanted to know how Prednisone and Cyclosporin made people diabetic. He said that was a "Nobel-prize winning question." Nobody understood the process. He then took me to Elizabeth's office where she went over the details with me.

Elizabeth explained to me the process of carbohydrate counting. Carbohydrates were broken down in the blood by insulin, a hormone. Carbs included breads, fruits and vegetables, pastas, cereals, grains, simple sugars like desert, and milk. If I consumed any of those things, I needed to count the number of carbohydrates in each serving. Nutrition labels on food packages would tell how much was in each serving. I could also buy a book that would list the content of most foods. After counting the number of Carbs, I would apply a formula to the total: divide by four. If breakfast contained one hundred grams of carbohydrate, my total insulin dose would be twenty five units of Humalog. I could also use Humalog to lower my glucose if it was high. Each unit of Humalog would lower my glucose by twenty points. If my glucose was one hundred and seventy, then I would subtract one hundred and thirty. The remainder, forty, would be divided by twenty. So I should take two units of Humalog. We used one hundred and thirty because that was almost in the upper normal glucose range of one hundred and twenty.

Dr. Buse and Elizabeth both stressed the importance of giving myself a shot right before I was about to eat. That way, my glucose would not rise too high before the insulin began to chew it up.

Within a week, my glucose ran mostly in the one hundred range. I was jubilant. My formulas needed a little tweaking and I would coordinate with Elizabeth. Instead of dividing by four, divide by five and add two. Instead of subtracting by one thirty and dividing by twenty, divide by fifteen. Scared by Dr. Egan's admonitions, I did not want to adjust my dose without talking with Elizabeth. But soon, she gave me permission to adjust my dose without checking with her.

Three weeks from my initial consult with Endo, my glucose ran within the normal range almost every time I checked it. It has remained virtually normal and in control ever since.

***

Normalcy began seeping back into my existence.

One night, a friend from college was in town so we all went out for seafood. Again, we went through our "no uncooked vegetables" routine. Again, my soft shell crabs came draped with fresh parsley. Karen urged me to send my dinner back, but I was hungry so I just removed it from my plate.

A few days later, we bumped into some new neighbors and struck up a conversation. I had only spoken with Jonathan twice before. On this occasion, he told us that they were on their way to see the Durham Bulls minor league baseball team. Had we ever been? I said that we were thinking about going, but I was having a hard time convincing Karen, who was not a huge baseball fan. The only way to get her to go to a game was to lure her with the promise of cotton candy. The next morning, Jonathan stopped by and said that he bought two extra tickets for that night's game. He was very handsome and gregarious, and that proved enticing enough that we did not have to mention any confectionery to Karen. We had a great time, eating hot dogs, watching very bad baseball, and making a few new friends.

***

Right around that time, a young woman asked me out. Beth was a pastoral counselor and a Baptist minister who helped people deal with grief. I could not think of a more unlikely person for a Yankee Jew like me to date, but thought that it would be interesting. She grew up in small Florida town outside of Tampa and had gone to college in Georgia. Consequently, she had a Southern accent. She was an avid white water rafter and water skier. And she was prone to expressions like "ripped me a new one."

Beth and I went out for coffee on Franklin Street. She wore no makeup, but she didn't need it. Almost immediately, we spoke about death. I was surprised that we could get into such a deep conversation without knowing each other too well. But she was fascinating.

She told me that when people were recovering from transplant, they were incredibly honest. They were stripped down to their core, unclouded by false airs. They were real. That was something she really liked about them.

***

Towards the end of June, my PFTs began to vacillate up and down just enough to raise Judy's eyebrows. She feared that it might be a sign of rejection so she asked me to come in and see the doctors. Clinic was not scheduled that day so she asked me to come right to the transplant office. Dr. Aris and a pulmonary fellow, Dr. Sunnuti, gave me a checkup. They could not decide whether or not I should get a bronchoscopy to determine if I was or was not in rejection.

Dr. Aris and Dr. Sunnuti then did something that I had never seen doctors do. They were indecisive about what action to take. So they asked Judy what she thought they should do. She said that they should bronch me. They agreed.

When I went in for my bronch this time, we made sure that I was completely isolated from the other patients. The hospital brass had explained that they were renovating Day-Op, but until that was completed, they instructed us to request isolation. Nobody wanted a repeat of the TB scare from the previous month.

There are two types of rejection, acute and chronic. Chronic rejection means that the lungs are slowly losing pulmonary function over a long period of time. It cannot be treated. Acute rejection means that the loss of pulmonary function is short-term and can be reversed with a high dose of steroids. With the bronch, my biopsies indicated mild acute rejection. It was completely normal and to be expected. Once again, the doctors put me on Solu-medrol for three days and Atavan for eight to prevent seizures.

CHAPTER 18

Returning Home to Maryland

I recovered quickly from my episode of rejection. It did, however, have one strange side effect. The combination of high dose steroids and Atavan thrust me into a funk for a week. I felt like Darth Vader wandering the halls of the Death Star. Surprisingly, nobody noticed. When I told my family and friends later on that I had been mildly depressed, they were shocked because I had appeared so normal.

One morning in rehab, Michael, Mary Ellen, and Nanette told me that we were allowed to go home for the Fourth of July weekend. It would be my first time back. I checked with Judy to see if it were true. For some reason, I was like the guy in the FedEx commercial, the last to know.

I got very excited at the thought of going home. We were cleared to leave Chapel Hill after rehab on Wednesday before the Fourth of July weekend. On Tuesday morning, I had to go to clinic in the ACC. There I saw Dr. Paradowski and Judy. After a check up, I asked if I could speak to Dr. Paradowski alone for a few minutes. Judy left the windowless exam room. Once we were alone, I thanked Dr. Paradowski for taking such good care of me throughout my transplant. I also thanked her for not doubting that I would pull through. We hugged and then talked about hockey.

Right after clinic, Mom, Bogart, and I left Chapel Hill. I was so anxious to go home that I skipped rehab on Wednesday. I had privately told Angie that I would be leaving Tuesday and promised to workout in Maryland.

That weekend, my friends enveloped me and I returned a conquering hero. Amy, Chuck, Simpson, Hefter, Taylor, Copperman, Katherine, Eve, Caroline and Mary all took me out for Vietnamese food. Decent Asian food at last. It tasted so good. I had been able to be apart from my friends, but seeing them made me realize how much I missed them. After dinner, we all went back to my house so that Mom and Dad could see everyone. They always joked that they missed my friends more than they missed me when I moved away.

Dr. Chernick and her husband, Sidney came over with an enormous Carvel ice cream cake. We all sat by the pool and I could see how proud she was. Ian also came over. Once again, he continued his mentorship, detailing things that I should expect. He told me that at the one year mark, the body chemistry settles down.

All weekend, Karen kept asking people: "Do you wanna see his scar?" Most people politely nodded. I would lift my shirt up, and bare all. They were grossed out for the most part. Being sensitive to market forces, I told Karen that we should hold off on show-and-tell.

I donned my wetsuit once again and swam in our pool every day. I also ate way too much. It was all high sodium and I was very bad. I gained six pounds and an extra chin.

The transplant team viewed our weekend away as a test. Would we page them every five minutes or would we be able to survive without them? I vowed that I would not need to call, and it worked out well. I proved my independence to them.

The weekend flew by, and on Sunday, we packed up the car and drove back to Chapel Hill. We sat in traffic for an hour and did not arrive until late at night. The apartment had its share of centipedes scurrying about and Mom went crazy eradicating them.

The Monday morning after I returned to Carolina, I bumped into Betty at the hospital. I had not seen her since we met at Eckerd pharmacy. As usual, she looked stunning, only now, she had added a rich, Hawaiian Tropic tan to the mix. We talked about the holiday and she told me that she shared a cabin with a girlfriend, water skiing and jet skiing on a lake somewhere in Carolina. It sounded like a perfect weekend, and I wished I had been there with her.

I would be allowed to move home permanently on July eighteenth. That was in just two weeks. Before that, a major milestone would arrive: the three month mark. That was the point at which I could eat fresh fruit, vegetables, and black pepper once again. For most of that time, the sacrifice had not been difficult. Once in a while, I would watch someone eat a salad with envy, but did not have major cravings. Some of my friends went nuts. By the end of their wait, they were beside themselves, dying for a salad. Ian, who never ate salad before his transplant, became obsessed with them. He has since consumed many.

The one food I especially looked forward to was a giant-sized Italian cold cut sub with everything from Jersey Mike's. I had not eaten there since the night of my last hockey game. One day I mentioned to Judy how much I was looking forward to that. She told me that the rule was three months after I left the hospital, which would put me back at July 30. I explained that it wasn't a feasible date because I would already be home in Maryland by then. Jersey Mike was in Chapel Hill, not Bethesda. Luckily, she conceded and allowed me to go there my last day in Carolina.

The temperature rose into the nineties that day and the sun beat down hard. We packed up two cars, and before heading out of town, paid a visit to Jersey Mike. I ordered my favorite, and it tasted just as I remembered it: a freshly baked sub roll perfectly complimented by premium meats and toppings. The memory is so powerful that I am salivating as I write this passage.

Before we left Chapel Hill, life was hectic. I continued to date Beth. We went to art galleries, coffee houses, dinner, and movies. Late one night after seeing the Disney adaptation of Hercules, I dropped her off at her house and we kissed goodnight. My first kiss with new lungs. Illuminated by the yellow light outside her door, she gave me the most beautiful smile.

I made the rounds and said goodbye to everyone. It was hard to leave Judy. One morning after Rehab, we shared a cup of coffee together in the outdoor picnic area underneath the cafeteria. She went over my upcoming schedule, when she wanted me to come back for a follow up, when I would receive my next doses of CytoGam; and how she should coordinate my care with my doctor up in Maryland. Then I gave her a gift, a sculpture of an Egyptian cat in white alabaster. The pose of the cat captured Judy's spirit.

Saying goodbye to Annette and Jay proved difficult. We had grown so close over the year, and they had been so kind to me. We planned to go to a Durham Bulls game with Mom and Dad but on the night in question, it was just too hot to sit outside for three hours. So we went out to a Greek restaurant in Durham. Annette marveled at how my parents still flirted with each other after more than thirty years of marriage.

At rehab, I said goodbye to Angie. I gave her a gift certificate for disco dancing lessons. Now she could finally learn the Hustle. To Annie, I gave a copy of my Mom's latest book, *The Angry American.*

I still had not heard back from Subaru regarding the poster that I wanted to sign and hang on the wall in rehab. To this day, the president of the company has not responded. Annie asked me to present a lecture to a class of physical therapy students. She asked me to describe the process of rehab for transplant. I put on a jacket and tie and met her in rehab. None of my Fighting Fivesome friends had ever seen me dressed up before. Nanette gave me an especially hard time, with Mary Ellen a close second. When I began my talk, I described my initial concerns about rehab: that it might take away from all of my other sports activities, and that I might not be able to go very long on the Stairmaster. It was the first time Annie had ever heard me say them, and she laughed.

On the bronchoscopy front, the hospital did an about-face about supporting our request for isolation. The administrators told us that isolation was not necessary and that they could not provide it. I was very upset about this, and made my concern loud and clear. I did not want isolation just for me, but for all transplant recipients. Dr. Paradowski called me up and promised that they would never do anything to harm me. I did not need isolation, but could request "segregation" at Day-op. If that was good enough for Dr. Paradowski, then it was fine with me.

I went to clinic one last time. There, Dr. Egan gave me a lecture on the importance of compliance. He said that some people start feeling good and decide that they don't need to follow the protocol. That's when they start having major problems. I knew that would not happen to me.

I had a few questions for him. Soon after I moved home, I planned to get a job. Would it be safe to ride the subway? Our family had been debating the pros and cons of public transportation being immuno-compromised. Dr. Egan joked that it was safe as long as I didn't get mugged.

Michael, Mary Ellen, Nanette and I went to support group one last time. Once again, we described for people waiting what life was like with new lungs. Then a young woman who had just gone on the waiting list and not yet moved down asked a question. "How do you keep from going crazy after you move down?" One person who had moved down and was still waiting gave the following answer: "Your life revolves around rehab. Not much else." I respected her answer. After all, some people are too sick to do too much else. My experience, though, had been different. "Continue to pursue the same things you were interested in back home. For me, I liked ice-hockey so I found a team down here. I liked writing so I joined the local chapter of Sisters in Crime. If you make your life revolve solely around rehab, you will be unhappy."

On my last weekend in Carolina, a huge group of us went out to the Macaroni Grill one last time. As usual, it was a great mix of transplant recipients, people waiting, physical therapists, and our family members. Dad had just flown in from Washington and he arrived with Mom right from the airport.

Charity and I went out for Indian food. Although her transplant had occurred the previous September, her health problems persisted. The transplant team felt that she needed to stay in Chapel Hill so that they could keep a close eye on her. Charity had to move there permanently. She missed her life in Florida, but accepted the team's request.

July was a difficult month for the transplant program. They lost four patients. I knew three of them. Two people were waiting. One was a teenager from Northern Virginia, Emil. He and I had shared many of the same respiratory therapists before I got the vest. The second was Teresa. She had asked the question in support group about how we kept from going crazy. The third person that I knew was a young man named Greg. He had worked for IBM and loved playing basketball. He was quite tall but very thin. He had been in and out of the hospital all winter and spring. One day, I bumped into him just outside of rehab. He sat in a wheelchair as he waited to be taken back up to his room. While he waited, he pored over his medical chart. It cracked me up and I gave him a hard time about it. Actually, it was something we all did, but with discretion. He was brazen. Greg had been extremely sick before his transplant. When he finally received it, he simply did not have the bodily reserves left to fight and recuperate.

The fourth patient I did not know. After they died, the members of the transplant team were visibly upset. They tried to conceal it around us, but by now, we knew them all very well. As with family members, I cannot imagine what they go through. Sometimes, it pains us to know that they are upset and not be able to comfort them.

Before we moved home, Dr. Yankaskis took Mom and me on a tour of the CF research lab at UNC. The lab was located in the Thurston-Bowles building, partly named after Skipper Bowles, Erskine's father. It sat just up the hill from the main hospital, near the ACC.

Dr. Yankaskis met us in his tiny, cramped office. Everybody was busily putting together a grant proposal, and the timing of our visit seemed poor. But Dr. Yankaskis dropped everything and proceeded to give us a tour that rivaled Willy Wonka's tour of his Chocolate Factory. He led us from room to room, explaining the research as we went. Like the Chocolate Factory, there was so much to see and not enough time to see it. His energy was limitless, his enthusiasm infectious. This very thoughtful, modulated man sprang to life as he spoke, his eyes bulging, his words speeding.

Dr. Boucher and Dr. Knowles took time out of their work to say hello and explain what they were up to. They wanted to know what my new lungs felt like.

Dr. Yankaskis pointed out a liquid nitrogen cooler stuck in one dark alcove. A pair of heavy duty gloves lay on top of it. My old lungs were stored inside for research. We walked away from our visit awed. We walked away grateful that these brilliant men and women dedicated their lives to CF. And we walked away feeling that the research breakthroughs could not come fast enough.

CHAPTER 19

Regaining a Normal Life

Returning to Maryland meant reconnecting with my former life. My health became less and less of an issue. No longer did I lead an isolated existence. No longer did I stay home by myself for most of the day. Now I was out, constantly meeting new people. My Sisters-in-Crime date book, which had held scant entries, now overflowed. I could not fit all of my activities into the space allowed. I felt myself circulating through society once again. Now my life was filled with vitality and stimulation.

One night, Jon Hefter took me to a party with his MBA friends. It was held on the rooftop of an apartment building in Kalorama, a neighborhood in Washington that included many embassies. The weather was warm, the sky was clear, and from our vantage point, we could see all of Washington and Northern Virginia lit up and glimmering. I looked around at the young, beautiful faces, and the spectacular skyline, smelled the rich scent of beer wafting out of large plastic cups, and felt immense gratitude. I was very lucky to be there.

In the ensuing months, I regained a sense of normalcy which I had not felt in years. I could go out and participate in one activity, and another and another, where before I could only really do one thing in an entire day. The sense of being sub-human dissolved.

I saw all of my friends. Rachel Burnett and I went out for lunch at the Cheesecake Factory. She was busy planning her fall wedding. One of the worst parts of living in North Carolina had been deserting my friends when they needed me. I was so glad that I was home and could go to her wedding in October.

As I began to swirl through civilization, I began to gauge a number of different reactions when I told people that I had undergone a transplant. Some people could not contain their happiness for me. A number of people were impressed and inspired. Others could not help dropping their jaw. The news was completely unexpected. Another group offered a grotesque sympathy. "Oh, what you must have been through," they would say, and shake their heads. Some people said: "How scary!" And a final group did not want to talk about it at all. That was fine with me. I understood that it must be fairly intense. For the most part, people fell under the 'ecstatic' category.

I reconnected with The Heat. Summer league was in full swing and I went to see them play. My teammates greeted me warmly and invited me to stand behind the bench for the game. For the rest of the summer, I went to all of their games and cheered them on. Like my return to the IcePlex in Raleigh, it was hard to watch and not participate. Judy still did not want me to even skate, much less play hockey, so I would have to wait.

By strange irony, the week after I moved home, the transplant team changed a policy. No longer would patients have to adhere to our strict diet. The no fresh fruit/ vegetables or black pepper rule would only be in effect while people were still in the hospital. Once home, they could eat anything they wanted. The transplant team found that the risk of Aspergillus was too remote to merit the constraint.

***

Due to the high doses of Prednisone and Neoral, my acne raged. The transplant team had given me medication to treat it, but it was ineffective. I scheduled an appointment with Dr. Samuel Norvell, my dermatologist.

Dr. Norvell explained to me that for Prednisone-related acne, a drug called Retin-A is the best possible treatment. He put me on it and it helped. I wished that I had begun my Retin-A treatment one week after my transplant when my chest broke out ferociously. It would have made me much more comfortable.

Dr. Norvell took a look at my chest tube scars and noticed that they had become "keloid." That meant that my scar tissue had built up excessively. He recommended a new treatment to alleviate the condition. Laura Ferris in Colorado and Judy had both suggested that I use vitamin E. But Dr. Norvell prescribed Epi-derm, a patch of silicon gel that would be taped over my chest tube scars. It worked incredibly well and again, I wished that I had begun using it much earlier.

***

The first weekend in August, Ian had a party to celebrate his one year anniversary. It was a joyous occasion and I was glad that I moved home in time to share it. Many of Ian's friends came, including some from as far away as Arizona. His parents and sister were there. His daughter, Ashley, led the way in demolishing a pinata that hung from a tree in the back yard. Linda, a former nurse of ours, came. She was a competitive body builder and trained with Ian in the gym. Michael Boyd, who had undergone a transplant two years ago, came with his wife.

They had just moved into a new home and it looked great. Ian proudly showed me his plans for the basement. It would include a sectional La-Z-Boy sofa and a wide screen TV so that everyone could fully enjoy watching the Redskins.

Ian's life was now smooth sailing. He had been so sick that he hung on to life by his fingernails before his transplant. Now he walked tall. He was a living testament to the power of medicine.

**

In early August, our family went up to Cape Cod. I flew to Boston and spent a night with Karen at her apartment. She threw a party for me and invited all of her friends. The women were all beautiful and one of them, Michelle, even played my crazy sport. The next morning, it was off to Wellfleet.

As we crossed over the Cape Cod Canal, I rolled down my window and breathed in the sweet air with my new lungs. It tasted just fine, only now I tasted much more of it.

It was great to do all of the things that I used to do on the Cape only with new lungs. Karen and I went sailing in Wellfleet Harbor. Dad and I played golf at Chequessett. We had linguica pizza at Rookies. And we went to Provincetown.

When we returned from the Cape, Dad and I went to Baltimore to see the Orioles. It was great to be back in Camden Yards Stadium with new lungs. This time, I did not cough. When we drove home, I was not exhausted. Before my transplant, I would always sleep during the forty-five minute drive back to Bethesda. This time, I drove. When we arrived home, I did not have to begin my routine with my nebulizer and vest.

**

Labor Day weekend, my family threw a huge welcome home party for me. We called it a "Blow the House Down" party. Mom and I made invitations that featured the wolf from the childrens' story "The Three Little Pigs" blowing hard. Aaron and Leslie Roffwarg flew up from

Houston for the weekend of the party to help us celebrate. Karen came down from Boston.

We had saved Amy's decorations from her "New Lung Shower" and hung them up. We bought a ton of deli platters. We bought plenty of beer. We heated the pool up. We were ready to go.

Over 150 people came that evening to eat and hang out by our pool. Almost all of my friends came. My old buddies from high school. Some members of the Heat. My Melrose Place gang. Ian Ferguson and Suzanne Tomlinson. Karen's friends. Mom and Dad's friends. Dr. Chernick. Bob Beall and his wife, Mimi. My old therapist, Joe Hamilton. Rachel and her fiancé, Evan. Our relatives and neighbors. It was a great mix and everyone had fun. The only trouble was that every time Jon Lastuvka and I tried to swap wild stories, we were interrupted. Other than that, it was a blast.

***

Early in September, my PFTs again went slightly erratic. Judy asked me to come down for a bronchoscopy. Now, life was in full swing for all of us and coordinating the trip would be difficult. I had a job interview at one of the best ad agencies in Washington. I did not want to miss it, but my parents were both back at work and could not take me any other time. I could not go down alone because I would be receiving anesthesia. Luckily, an old friend of mine from high school, Phil Saltzman, was on shore leave from the merchant marine.

I called Phil up and asked him if he'd like to go on a road trip. Sure, he replied. When did I want to leave? In an hour.

"No problem." There was just one catch. "Could we stop just north of Richmond to see a girl?"

"Absolutely." I really appreciated his friendship.

We had a good time on that trip. Phil took a crash course in transplant, learning all about its intricacies. We talked about lots of things on the drive down and back. We went out for barbecue in Chapel Hill. And we stayed in the Hampton Inn. I had not been there since before moving the past December.

Phil seemed nervous that I might be sick. He was also interested in the medicine. He served as "ship's doctor" when he was at sea, treating sick crew members until they could be med-evacced to shore.

After my bronch, he snuck out to Jersey Mike's and bought me a giant-sized Italian cold cut sub. By the time I woke up from the sedation, it was mid-afternoon and I was starving. I had not eaten a thing since the night before. Halfway through the sub, my doctors came to recovery and caught me eating. They panicked, fearing that the anesthesia had not worn off from my throat and I could choke. I knew that I could swallow before I took a bite, so I chomped away.

Before leaving the hospital, I wanted to stop by Anderson Four and see a few people. A whole new class had received transplants within the past two weeks. Joanna, from New York. Jeff from Ohio. And Brett, who I had worked out with in rehab before mine.

Brett looked great when we saw him. He had withstood some digestive problems, but now felt much better. He was alert and in good spirits. Brett thanked me for a gift I had sent him. After hearing about his transplant, I followed the Julie Fanburg gift-giving guide and sent him *Playboy*'s "Girls of the Big Ten Conference" edition. Brett's recovery was so strong that he ended up putting the rest of us to shame. He actually drove himself home from the hospital. And he went back to work four weeks after his operation. I still don't know how that is possible.

Phil and I met Jeff. His transplant had occurred just two days earlier. He was already out of the ICU and progressing famously. He was sitting up, conversant, and very cheery. I know that he must have been happily stoned, but it did not show. I did not look anywhere near that good two days after mine.

Phil had two reactions to seeing Brett and Jeff. He found them very inspiring. He said that meeting them was worth the price of the entire trip. He also was struck by how much we sounded like physicians when we spoke, conferring about medications, dosing, and treatments.

My bronch showed another bout of mild-acute rejection. Judy asked me to come down in two weeks for a clinic check up. They put me on Solu-medrol and I went in for that job interview with an IV in my arm.

For the follow-up visit to Carolina, I drove myself down. On the way, I stopped in Richmond to see my friends at Circuit City. I had not been back to my old office since I was forced to leave four years earlier. Many of my former co-workers were still there, and it was great to see them. The company's prosperity was obvious. Where before the corporation was housed in one building, now there were three. Since my departure, they had added an entire new division, CarMax, devoted to selling used cars. Business was booming.

At clinic the next day, I met with two new physicians. They told me that my blood showed a new development: my antibodies had converted for Epstein-Barr virus. Conversion after transplant meant that I was now at a thirty percent higher risk for contracting lymphoma. That scared the heck out of me. They assured me that it was very treatable and I should not be concerned. They asked that once a week, I feel my armpits, groin, and neck for anything unusual. That way they could catch it early.

To reduce the risk of lymphoma, they would have to change the dosing of my meds. Cyclosporin would be lowered and Prednisone would be raised. The raising of my Prednisone frustrated me. I had gotten my dose down to the lowest it had ever been, 17.5 mgs. By November, it was scheduled to be minuscule, 15mgs every other day. Now, I was right at the threshold where the side effects would be minimal. My diabetes might even go away. That had happened to Brian Urbanek and Tom Faraday when their Prednisone tapered down. Now, I would need to keep it relatively high all the way until my one year anniversary, thereby postponing the reduction in side effects. Thereby postponing the possibility that my diabetes might abate.

During that visit, UNC ran a follow up bone density scan. It showed no change from immediately after my surgery. I had been sure that the high doses of steroids would have chewed up my bones.

I asked the doctors and Judy one last question. My PFT's were now strong. My FVC was 4.0 and my FEV1 was at 3.3. How much longer would they continue to rise? Judy answered. She said that the numbers would go up until the sixth month mark. I had one more month. In mid-October, when that anniversary fell, I got a little depressed at the thought that my numbers would not rise any higher. Actually, I proved them wrong. My numbers continue to rise, even to the one year mark, at this writing. My FEV1 is now 3.8, over 100 percent.

Ian told me that his numbers continue to rise, more than a year and a half after his transplant. He says that exercise is a huge factor in expanding his new lungs.

✱✱✱

Once again, my life proceeded at full swing. I began dating ferociously, like I had never dated before. Each weekend, I went out with a different woman. A lawyer. A junior high school teacher. A psychologist. The manager of a hospice. A saleswoman. Beth had moved up from North Carolina to work at a church in Northern Virginia. We went out.

In September, I reunited with the Chesapeake chapter of Sisters in Crime. At a luncheon featuring a speech by a local forensic archeologist, the sisters all welcomed me home and made a big fuss. They had not changed a bit, and still pursued fascinating topics like hostage negotiation and corporate espionage. It was great to be back.

I went back to the JCC to begin working out there again. I didn't lift weights yet, but did work out on the treadmill, and a wonderful new machine, the Reebok Body Trek. It simulated cross-country skiing. The only difference between this and rehab was that now there was nobody to place a fan in front of me or pop CDs in a stereo. I had to buy a small Walkman and be a disc jockey for myself.

In October, I hit the six month mark and Judy let me resume two of my passions, weight lifting and ice-hockey. I started weight lifting first to build my upper body up for hockey. Then I started skating. Hitting the ice again felt good, but my legs had a long way to go. My skating was off, as was my balance and leg strength.

Two weeks later, hockey season began. I was able to consummate the thoughts that had obsessed me since the ICU. Now I would find out what it felt like to play with normal, healthy lungs. On my very first shift, I skated hard and fast. When I got back to the bench two minutes later, I was not out of breath. For the entire game, I did not get winded. Evinrude was gone. My lungs worked great.

My game day routine was very different from before my transplant. Now I did not need to do all of my chest PT before hand. Now I did not need to rush home and do a neb treatment after the game. I did not need to scarf down high-salt pretzels. It was strange, but I was glad.

My legs could not keep up with my lungs. They were racked by terrible shin splints. The pain was agonizing, almost to the point of tears. By the end of the game, I could barely stand. But I wanted to play so badly. I called Annie Downs and Ian Ferguson, asking for advice. Annie suggested that I ice my shins down before and after each game. That helped. She also explained that the problem might be "compartmentalization syndrome," where the muscles in front of my shin bones had nowhere to expand. The calves in comparison, could grow and swell as much as they needed to. When she explained that to me, I decided to try something new. Normally, I would tape my shin pads down very tight. Maybe that added to the compartmentalization. I tried not taping them down at all. That gave the muscles more room and it helped reduce the pain. Ian recommended some exercises to build up the strength in my shin muscles. Judy told me that I might be depleting my body of magnesium. Before my games, I made sure to take a magnesium pill and that helped immensely.

Sometimes I missed North Carolina. In the eight months that I lived there, I did not hear the term "road rage" used once. In Washington, it made the news every week. I missed the friendliness of North Carolina, of strangers who hugged you in a furniture rental store, or neighbors who invited you to a minor league baseball game. I felt like Crocodile Dundee when he visited New York. As he walked down the street in the Big Apple, he tipped his hat and said "Goodday" to every passerby who looked at him as if he were a freak.

***

I checked myself regularly in the armpits, groin and neck, and everything felt normal. My insomnia, which had gone away soon after I got out of the hospital, resumed in mid October. It was very frustrating so I called the transplant team. Judy was away so I spoke with Jean. She suggested that instead of taking my Prednisone in two doses, with breakfast and dinner, I take all of it at dinner. That did the trick. My insomnia went away. Sometimes, I got terrible night sweats. Judy said that it was probably from the Epstein-Barr virus conversion.

Otherwise, I felt very good. I could feel myself getting stronger and stronger. In the gym, my weightlifting was progressing well. I began doing squats and using free weights. I had been using machines because Dr. Rosenstein felt that the intense exertion from free weights put me at a high risk for a collapsed lung. Now I could grasp the steel free weights once again.

Two momentous events happened in November. Julie Perlmutter hired me to help her work for an advertising agency, McCann-Erickson. She was a consultant to the Washington office. The work was part time, but I loved it. It felt great to once again be enmeshed in the world of advertising.

The second event occurred at the National Institutes of Health. The NIH broke ground on a new clinical research facility and asked me to give a speech at the ceremony.

Before my speech, Mom, Dad, Karen and I attended a private reception. There Karen and I spoke with Dr. Francis Collins, the head of the Human Genome Project. Dr. Collins is a true legend in the CF community. He was one of three men who discovered the CF gene. Dr. Collins is very tall and unassuming. Like Dr. Paradowski, Dr. Chernick, and Dr. Rosenstein, he is a very modest person. With reddish blond hair and a thick mustache, Karen describes him as extremely handsome. In his spare time, he rides a Harley-Davidson motorcycle.

Dr. Collins asked me the same question that Dr. Boucher and Dr. Knowles asked: how did my transplant affect my life? I gave my usual response: no coughing, no five hours a day of chest PT.

Then Karen interjected. "Oh no. He's giving you the official, censored answer. Do you want the unofficial, unabridged version?"

Dr. Collins nodded enthusiastically.

"He's dating all over the place. He's got breakfast dates. He's got lunch dates. He's got dinner dates. He goes dancing. He plays ice-hockey. He's making an overprotective sister like me very nervous."

We all broke up laughing.

In my speech, I called the new Mark Hatfield Clinical Research Center a "living shrine to my heros," NIH scientists. I catalogued all of the medical advances in CF that NIH had helped fund. Along with the CF Foundation, NIH helped pay for the discovery of the gene. NIH helped pay for the introduction of Pulmozyme. It helped pay for the development of the Flutter. It helped pay for advances in life-saving antibiotics like Ciprofloxacin and nebulized Tobramycin. I described how I had been affected by each of those advances.

***

On the Wednesday before Thanksgiving, I conducted my routine lymphoma check. This time, I flunked. I felt a small lump under my right chest muscle. I called Dr. Pollack and rushed right over to see him thirty minutes later. He felt it and said that he did not know what it was. I would need to have it biopsied. With me in his office, he called up Judy and discussed the matter with her. She agreed that it should be biopsied as soon as possible. Biopsy was a word I did not want to get involved with. He referred me to a local surgeon. I thought I was through with those people.

Over the weekend I felt the bump each day and was convinced it grew. The following Monday, I saw the surgeon, Dr. Hanowell. He studied the bump and determined that it needed to be biopsied. He scheduled me for the following morning. I did not want to panic my family. After all, they had been through enough. So I did not mention any of this to them. There was still a chance that it could be nothing at all. If it were cancer, then I would tell them.

The next morning, I drove myself to the surgical center. Dr. Hanowell used lidocaine to numb the entire area and that is all I felt. I had not asked him for anything to help me relax, partly so that I could drive myself, and partly because I did not need it. The lump was directly underneath my transplant incision so he cut right through that in a one centimeter portion. He was very skilled and the new incision was not noticeable.

I asked him how soon I could play hockey again. He told me to wait two hours. "Great" I replied. I happened to have a game that night that I did not want to miss. That took him aback. He did not expect me to play so soon. He told me to put extra padding over the bandage. In a week, the steri-strip would peel away on its own. The sutures were under the skin and would dissolve on their own. I called Judy and asked her if I could take Tylenol if I were in pain. She said that was fine. I ended up not needing it. And I played very well that night. My new incision stayed sutured shut even when I hit a few opponents pretty hard.

A week later, I received good news about the biopsy. It was benign: fat that had lost its supply of blood. Like the rabbi who plays golf on the Sabbath and scores a hole-in-one, I could not share my good news with anyone. That was okay. I was deeply grateful. Judy knew and it was good to be able to talk about it with her.

★★★

That Saturday, I made my debut in the world of professional sports. Abe Pollin followed through on a promise he made a year earlier. His new sports palace, the MCI Center opened up in the beginning of December in downtown Washington. He gave us a tour not unlike the way Dr. Yankaskis showed us around his lab. Abe is a self-described "sports freak" and the building reflected that side of his personality. There was an interactive sports museum where you could shoot hoops against the Wizard's star, Chris Webber.

The Washington Capitals dedicated their inaugural game to me and I dropped the ceremonial puck. I skated out onto the ice, shook hands with Dale Hunter, the Caps' Captain, and Scott Mellanby, Captain of the Florida Panthers. Then I let the rubber fly.

It was great fun and the Capitals won in overtime.

★★★

In early January, Karen and I went West. My parents generously teamed up with some family friends, Harold and Jonny Kozupsky, to send us skiing for a week in Utah. We stayed in Salt Lake City and skied at all of the surrounding resorts: Alta, Park City, Deer Valley, and Snowbird. Karen could not keep up with me. I wanted to ski all day and now my lungs and legs allowed me to do just that. When Karen struggled to keep up, she realized that now she did not have to worry about my health any more.

I recalled the e-mail I received from Laura Ferris. She had told me that on her ten-month anniversary, she was on her honeymoon, jet skiing in the Bahamas. Now I was at my nine month, schussing through two feet of fresh powder. It was awesome.

We ate like pigs, steak and Tex-Mex almost every night. We scoped like crazy. And we made plenty of new friends. On our last night, we went to the Sundance Film Festival.

This was a trip I would not have dared to venture on prior to my transplant, even when I was healthier. The altitude of 10,000 feet contained much less oxygen, and would have made breathing too difficult. Now, I went to that elevation and did not feel a thing. No dizziness, no shortness of breath. None of the symptoms that even perfectly healthy people sometimes suffer.

Before flying home from Utah, I received a phone call from Dr. Yankaskis. He was planning this year's "Evening With the Master Chefs." Last year's event took place on the night of my transplant. Would I like to come and speak this year? Heck yes. It would be April nineteenth. I called up Amy Kingman, who I had planned to take a year ago. "Remember that rain check?" I asked her. She was free and looked forward to the dinner.

In March, I finally bought a poster for rehab. After giving up on Subaru, I moved on to hockey. At first, I wanted to buy a poster of Washington Capital's star Peter Bondra. I could not find one. Then I wanted a poster of the US Women's Olympic hockey team. I had followed them closely and was elated when they won the gold. I couldn't find a poster of them either. Then I found a poster of Wayne Gretzky. It was the perfect image, one that could endure on the walls of rehab and inspire future generations of transplant recipients. It conveyed a positive spirit, emotion, and greatness.

***

In April, I celebrated my one year anniversary. To do so, I played ice-hockey. Then, Mom, Dad, Karen and I went out for a big steak dinner at Ruth's Chris Steak House.

Four days later, I had my seventh bronch. It was the last one that was scheduled. Now, the doctors would only perform the procedure if I had a problem. The following day, I went to clinic. In the waiting room, I saw Nanette for the first time since we moved away. She had been having problems, and the doctors were trying to figure out what was wrong. Despite not feeling well, she gave me a huge hug.

That morning, Dr. Paradowski and Judy gave me the early results of my bronch. There were no signs of rejection or infection. My lungs looked terrific.

Then Dr. Paradowski gave me the best news of all: I could taper down my Prednisone to a very low dose.

Before leaving clinic, Judy gave me a hand-held spirometer. She still wanted me to use my Datalog at home, but now when I traveled, I could bring this new device instead. The advantage was that it was very small, and light. It would make traveling a piece of cake. I was so happy that I told her this would now enable me to travel lighter than I had in fifteen years.

I stayed in North Carolina for the weekend, spending it with Annette and Jay. Sunday night, I attended the CF Foundation's fundraiser, "An Evening With The Master Chefs." This was the event that I missed the year before because of my transplant. Amy Kingman, who was supposed to go with me last year, kept her promise of a rain check and came one year later.

Dr. Yankaskis was there, as was Dr. Boucher, and Dr. Egan. Amy and I also had the opportunity to meet Howell Graham, the first CF patient that got new lungs at UNC. He looked amazing, full of beans, happily married to a gorgeous dentist, and successful in business. It was seven years since his transplant.

In my speech that night, I discussed the power of medicine. I told the audience that I was living proof that research worked. They each had the power to cure disease, and by attending the event, they exercised that power.

That June, I began to work full-time once again, for a large advertising agency, Bates USA. I have been working ever since. Now my advertising adventure has taken me to OgilvyInteractive, part of Ogilvy & Mather.

The Lessons of My Transplant

The most important lessons of transplant concern awareness and gratitude.

First for awareness. Wild Woman should not have had to wait forty months for her transplant. People in Boston should not have to wait three to five years. I should not have had to wait 28 months. Thousands of people die every year because a donor is not found in time to save them. This should not happen. Many people die after their transplants because they are very sick by the time they receive their new organs. This should not happen.

The severe shortage of organs can be significantly reduced. People need to tell their families that if they are ever in the position to donate their organs, they wish to do so. Merely signing an organ donor card does not necessarily mean that a person's wishes will be carried out. Family members are given the ultimate responsibility for fulfilling a loved one's wishes. The worst thing in the world is for a potential donor

to be available, but because his family does not know his wishes, his
organs go to waste.

One day last August, I navigated my shopping cart through the bak-
ery section of the local supermarket. There I bumped into Mitch Yanoff,
the owner of The Hockey Stop, a local hockey store. He remarked that
I hadn't been by the shop in a while. When I told him where I'd been,
he was floored, and very happy for me. Then he made a wonderful comment. "I'm so glad that you told me that because I'm about to go up to
the Motor Vehicle Administration to renew my driver's license. My wife
and I have been debating how to respond to the organ donor question.
Now I know." That was incredibly gratifying.

The next time your family sits down to eat dinner, initiate a dialogue.
After you say "Darling Nikki, please pass the ketchup," or "Aunt
Esmerelda, could you toss the salad?" then broach the subject of trans-
plant. Your conversation could save several lives.

We need to fund more research into transplantation to develop
alternative avenues for donation. New treatments could open the door
for whole new classes of donors. Currently, people who die of cardiac
failure cannot donate their organs. So many of them die in hospitals
that they would otherwise be ideal donors. If medicine figures out a
way to utilize their organs, it would virtually eliminate all waiting lists
and save many lives.

As Ellen Crabtree Brooks pointed out to us, "nobody wants to
become an organ donor, but if you are dead, you are done with your
organs. You simply do not need them anymore. At the same time, you
have the chance to save somebody else's life."

My donor and her family made that decision and it saved my life.
Transplant works. We have a responsibility to nurture this new medicine, to let it blossom, to let it save thousands of lives.

Now for the lesson of gratitude.

In our society, human life sometimes carries very little value. People
kill over a pair of sneakers or a traffic dispute. Transplant repudiates

that mentality. With transplant, life has an immense value. So many people work incredibly hard just to save one life.

I personally am grateful to the countless nurses, doctors, nutritionists, respiratory therapists, and physical therapists who all helped me.

I am grateful to my parents, sister, and grandmother who took me to all of those appointments; to Mom, Dad and Karen who sublimated their own anxieties, raced down to Chapel Hill at a moment's notice early one Sunday morning in April, and dropped their lives to stay with me for three months. To parents who offered emotional support, friendship, guidance, and financial aid over an entire lifetime. And I am grateful to a sister who doubled as a nurse.

I am grateful to friends who never treated me like a sick person; kept me connected to the world; and offered all of their support in my fight.

I am grateful to all the patients on whose broad shoulders I stand. They had the guts to pioneer transplant before there were any life expectancy numbers to rely on. The surgeons refined their techniques on them. The general medicine doctors learned on them. They stepped into the unknown and paved the way for people like me. Unlike the strength I found from the *Random Acts of Kindness* poem, these brave souls faced their transplants at a time when they did not know whether they would find something firm to stand on or if they would be taught to fly.

I am grateful to Blue Cross/ Blue Shield of the National Capital Area for paying for my transplant. That in itself was an enormous burden. When the letter for pre-approval came, our family heaved a sigh of relief. Twenty-eight months later, they followed through on their promise. Since then, they have paid over $200,000 on my care.

Finally, I am grateful to my donor, Val. She is a true hero.

***

Some lessons I have tried to tacitly convey. Most notably among them is the power of a positive mind set. I first learned it scurrying up and down the suburban soccer fields of Bethesda, listening to the upbeat encouragement of Mrs. Fisher. For many people this is unrealistic. When your whole body is racked with nausea from chemotherapy, it is hard to be upbeat about anything. I understand that, and think it is unfair to expect sunshine and cheerleading. There were days when I could not be positive. But for the most part, it helped me immensely.

So did the ability to fight. Fighting got me climbing the stairs of the NIH when I was in the hospital for IV treatments. Fighting got me to spend five hours a day on respiratory therapy. And fighting got me playing ice-hockey six days before my transplant. It paid off.

My perspective on fighting relates to the old adage about when life gives you lemons, make lemonade. My feeling has been, if life doesn't give you lemons, do what it takes to get them. Then make lemonade and market the hell out of it.

I cannot underscore enough the importance of pursuing one's interests. Temporarily abandoning my advertising career was difficult. But writing mysteries, dating beautiful women, eating Jersey Mike's Italian cold cut subs, playing "that sport," and keeping in touch with my friends helped maintain my sanity when I had nothing else to do but wait.

Remaining in control of one's self-definition is vital. Dad always told me: "You decide which girl you want to marry. You decide what career you want to have." That lesson applied to my health. I decided to define myself not as a sick person, but as an advertising executive, ice-hockey player, fundraiser, and writer. That definition is different from denying an illness. I do not urge people to disavow their health, but rather to address it head on and fight. And to not let it become the sole dimension to one's existence.

As Bob Simpson told me when I was sixteen, learning everything you can about your disease is very important. Because of the CF Foundation, Dr. Chernick and Dr. Rosenstein, I learned about CF.

Because of Trio, support group, and all of my friends who blazed a trail ahead of me, I learned about transplant.

Identifying positive role models is crucial. Arnold Schwarzennegger exemplified how beautiful muscles could look. Ian and Suzanne demonstrated successful marriage despite having CF. Karen proved that a young person could write a novel. Monica Goretski showed me how to be a successful recipient. In so doing, each of them helped me self-actualize.

One must learn to balance hypochondria with vigilance. Everything is completely new after transplant: the medicines, the diet, the routine. The chemistry of the body changes dramatically. At first, I did not know if excessive ear wax or large nipples were dangerous side effects. It is hard to know when to page the lung transplant coordinator on call. My friends and I have paged them at all hours of the night and interrupted every life activity imaginable. Slowly, one learns.

Slowly, one learns how to balance self advocacy with trust. To go through a transplant, a person must place complete trust in the entire team. I had to trust the physical therapists when they told me that rehab would be beneficial. I had to trust that Will was a good social worker even though we did not hit it off at first. I had to trust that even though I did not know who it would be, the surgeon would be very talented. I knew none of that for sure at the outset. On the flip side, no program is perfect. The UNC team was not able to treat my diabetes or acne. The hospital made a big mistake with my kidneys. And Day-Op exposed me to a dangerous risk of TB. We had to learn when to speak up and argue for change.

A Final Note

When I was first diagnosed with CF at the age of five, my life expectancy was eight. Now for a person with CF, it is 31. That number has risen throughout my lifetime due to the great strides in CF research.

The CF Foundation proved that good science can be bought. I am living proof that research works.

We have the power to cure disease. When your poker buddy says: "I'm raising money for Cancer research," offer to sponsor him. When the guy who works in the next cubicle over from you says that he's golfing to raise money for Sickle Cell Anemia, ask if you can lace up your cleats, dust off your clubs, and golf with him. When a dear friend develops lupus, take it upon yourself to find out how you can help.

We must foster the age of medicine for all diseases. We must challenge scientists to make more and more breakthroughs. And we must position them for success by providing the resources that they need.

The End

❀

About the Author

Charlie Tolchin lives in Washington, D.C., with his dog, Bogart. He works for OgilvyInteractive, a division of Ogilvy & Mather Advertising. For fun he plays ice-hockey, lifts weights and skis.

He can be contacted at: Blowthehousedown@aol.com

References

Cystic Fibrosis Foundation: Www.cff.org, 1-800-fight-CF
Transplant Recipients International Organization, TRIO: www.trioweb.org
United Network for Organ Sharing, UNOS: www.unos.org